Teresa Karr 6.95
45
—
7.40

Karen Kingston
P.O. Box 1189
Oceanside, CA 92054
e-mail clutter@spaceclearing.com

The Only Diet
There Is

To Linda,
You are very loved,
Teresa

D0049765

clutter @ spaceclearing.
com

The Only Diet There Is

Sondra Ray

Celestial Arts
Berkeley, California

Celestial Arts
P.O. Box 7327
Berkeley, California 94707

Cover design by Pat Goff
Typography by HMS Typography
Printed and bound by George Banta Company

First printing, October 1981
Manufactured in the United States of America

Library of Congress Cataloging in Publication Data

8 9 10   88 87 86 85 84

My greatest pleasure of all is dedicating this book
to you, Robert Rosellini, King of my cuisine.

Susan Ariel Rainbow Kennedy

You give me glorious feasts, fit for a saint,
      And I am spiritually nourished.
You take me beyond my limits of expansion,
      And I am exalted.
You fill me with the nectar of fire,
      And I become the breath inside the breath.
                  I love you.

I see your beauty,
      I feel your heart,
I taste your essence,
      I smell your bouquet,
I touch your soul,
      I hear your melody.

I drink of you at every breath.
I drink of the Divine.

Drawing adapted from a painting by Don Wyman

Contents

The Only Diet There Is

Food for Thought: Thought for Food

Preface by Fred Lehrman

Nourishment is certainly the least acknowledged of personal daily miracles. The alchemy of digestion and new cell formation is at the source of the life process itself. "Wonder Bread helps build strong bodies twelve ways"—this is indeed a wonder.

I have a friend who has completed a long experiment with diet. After growing to maturity on the average fare of a Brooklyn-born Columbia University student, he migrated to Idaho, where for one year he "took as many mind-altering drugs as possible." He made it through this test in fine shape. Then he went to a Zen monastary in California, where he became a monk and served as chief cook and gardener. For the first time in two years he followed a strict macrobiotic system, avoiding all sweets and red meat, gradually narrowing down to brown rice, salt plums, and a few cooked vegetables. His health was extremely good.

After almost three years of this, he suddenly switched to a diet consisting entirely of raw fruits and juice. From the macrobiotic point of view, this should have produced drastic and unpleasant effects on both mind and body. He still felt wonderful. In fact, the less he ate, the better he felt. He reached a point where for several months he would just chew one or two apples each day, swallowing only the juice and spitting out the meat. He found he could regulate his weight at will while on this diet, gaining or losing five pounds in a day, just by setting his mind on it. He continued this diet until winter, when he added some vegetables to keep his body warmer.

One day, while sitting with the other monks at their meal, he suddenly realized that he had been resisting his Zen practice by "discriminating" so much in his food choices. With that thought, he turned his inverted rice bowl right-side-up and received the monastery food he had refused for so long. Thereafter, he continued to accept as right for him whatever food he was offered. Later, he left the monastery and bought a farm in Northern California where he grew vegetables and raised livestock. His dinner table was set with whatever was ready to harvest on that day.

I asked him then what he had learned about "proper" diet. He paused a moment and said: "It's all a state of mind." His theory was that when one eats a carrot, for example, it isn't the cells of the carrot which transmute in our bodies to become living flesh. Based on his experience with the apples, he thought that the food we eat tunes our systems to a vibrational code. We then absorb pure life energy through breathing, and create new tissue as a direct process of thought. The carrot or apple serves as a catalytic aid. He mentioned to me that there are many documented cases of people like Theresa Neuman who have lived for years in a state of religious ecstacy without eating at all. Also, the findings of homeopathic medicine indicate that a remedy administered in a highly diluted form can have a more powerful effect than a massive dose of the same substance. Perhaps just thinking "carrot" in the right way could set in motion the same functions as are triggered when we actually eat one.

This book, *The Only Diet There Is*, addresses this premise, and offers a practical method which you can safely test for yourself. What we believe is what we experience; by changing our attitudes, our bodies will use our food differently. The proof of this pudding however, is still in the tasting. Try Sondra's diet. See what happens.

Sondra, I Salute You. . .

Preface by Linda Thistle, Ph.D., Psychotherapist-Rebirther

Driving up the California coast one glorious winter day, Sondra Ray read me the text of this book. It was stunning. Yet the message so simple, so true, I was amazed it hadn't been written before. I volunteered to be the first "subject," the first tried-and-tested "experiment." Would this really work? The next day I began this unusual diet. Life has never been quite the same. By the end of the week I'd lost several pounds, but more important I was so in love with life—and myself—I had the self-worth to create a beautiful body. Within one month I had lost 15 pounds, achieving my perfect body weight. And since I'm more powerful when I'm thin, there were other side-effects: an important relationship was healed; "Outrageous Woman," a convening of women committed to personal and global transformation, was successfully created and produced. Since then, I have recommended this "diet" to friends and clients. Many have tried it with dramatic results.

This, of course, is no ordinary "diet" book. Its subject is neither food nor eating. This is an extraordinary approach to weight loss—a "diet of forgiveness," a "fast from negative thought"—and if followed one can achieve bodily perfection.

The theory is simple. Though we might think it is our negative eating habits that have kept us unattractive and unhealthy, it is really our negative thoughts and feelings. It is the latter we must change for that is what is aging and killing us. If we do—if we forgive the past, drop negative thoughts and resentment, stop being victims—we drop our fat as well, for the same mechanism that holds on to negative thoughts and feelings holds on to fat. Releasing excess weight in our minds and hearts, we release excess weight in our bodies. Furthermore, all the energy of resentment—"resending" our thoughts, feeling, attention to a past that is not real any more—is a waste, an energy leak. When we drop resentment we release energy into the present. Since energy is an actual physical phenomenon flowing through our bodies, it burns calories, dissolves fat; we can begin to vibrate at our perfect body weight. Released from negativity we will be released from the overeating we've done to dull our guilt and grief and stuff our anger and hate. Released from self-pity self-loathing and blame, we will be released from the helplessness that has prevented us from mastering our bodies. We will be released from the bulk and bulges we think protect and pad us from past and possible present pain; we will be released from the constant, gnawing hunger that keeps us gobbling and gorging. We will be released from appetites never satisfied by food that does not and cannot nourish because our resistance, fear and resentment have blocked the experience of love. We will, at last, be full and free, fulfilled and satisfied.

The message of this book is transformative, not only physically and personally, but spiritually and socially. This is a critical time in human history. We have accumulated enough physical and metaphysical knowledge and tools to break continuity with the limitations of our past. We can, if we want, create a new human, a new age, a new world. We can create heaven on earth. But to do so we must render the past powerless through forgiveness. We can no longer use our relationships to hold us to the past. We can no longer afford to blame past circumstances, past failures, our parents, institutions, ourselves for our present condition. The same process, forgiveness and dropping our negative thoughts, which frees us from our past, frees us from our fears, frees us from our fat.

And how do we fantasize our possible paradise? Certainly not with dowdy, dumpy people, moaning about their bulges and groaning helplessly about their eating patterns. Oh no! We picture paradise peopled with prototypes of physical perfection. It is possible to become one of those perfect physical specimens if we master our present reality, for in the power and peace of the present we release our future, our perfect potential. Forgiveness releases energy into the Now, it releases us to do miracles now—this includes reshaping our bodies—into perfect health, perfect beauty, the perfect weight.

Sondra Ray IS a woman of the future. When I first saw her I blurted out, "Ohhhh, she's a goddess." She embodies the message of this book—tall, slim, shimmering with love and vitality. She not only looks perfect, she seems to have a certain genius to devise wise and simple techniques that help free us from our limitations.

Personally, using her suggestions and tools, musical gifts previously hidden were freed and are still flourishing; money, formerly a cause of great dread and discomfort, has become enormous fun and is much more abundant; and the anxiety, suffering and pain which too frequently stifled my life force and happiness, virtually disappeared. These are a few benefits of knowing Sondra. And of course, the message and techniques in this book continue to teach me mastery of my body. Sondra, I salute you, I love you, you've done it again. I recommend, without reservation, this book and Sondra to everyone.

There is no doubt the subject of this book will be of wide

interest. Every best-seller list seems to always include the latest diet book. However, this book is not just for those aspiring to their perfect body-weight. It is for everyone. For all of us long to lose the psychic, emotional and spiritual "weights" that have made us heavy in mind, heart and spirit.

So when this book is a #1 bestseller (and it should be) it could transform not only our bodies, but a nation and a world. For forgiveness restores the condition of unconditional love; it restores us to our true nature. We will be awakened as the gods we really are, physical and spiritual beauties, flowing with the sap, the juice, of unleashed love.

To My Friends

This book is about going all the way!

This book is not just about losing weight. Every truth in it can be used to heal all the other problem areas in your life.

You'll enjoy this book even if you are not trying to lose weight.

You'll enjoy this book even if you don't have a problem right now.

You'll enjoy your relationship with me while reading this book.

A spiritual diet is always enjoyable.

Love,

Sondra Ray!

Prologue

This book was started on a lovely, secluded old Cape Cod estate, the home of Lucy McRowell. The night before I began to write it, I was hanging out in the kitchen with my friends Bobby B. and Phil Laut. We shared what we had learned about weight from our consultations with clients.

Phil talked about the influence fashion models have on our ideas of female beauty. The first fashion models of women's clothing were very curvy, voluptuous women. These women had bodies that were getting more attention than the clothes! To end this problem, very slender, even skinny, women came to be chosen as models. These models got people to look at the clothes, rather than at the bodies in them. As a result, yesterday's female body type, chosen because it would be ignored, has become today's ideal!

"Here we are," I laughed, "going after something that is ridiculous, for the wrong reasons!"

Then I remembered how I often notice it is more fun to hug a woman who is soft and a little fleshy and voluptuous. In fact, I do not particularly like hugging a woman who is skinny and bony. *So why am I trying to be skinny and bony?* Am I wanting to be something less sensuous, possibly even unhealthy, because of messages from the media?

Phil also talked about something he had observed in watching babies. Babies are burped and then held right after they have eaten, when they have a full stomach. Therefore very early in life we get used to getting love when our stomaches are full! And we still have that link between food and love going on in our lives. This, I thought, was a very astute observation.

We also talked about a connection Phil had noticed between women who are overweight and women who have trouble saying *no* to men. It is fairly common knowledge by now that people put on weight to avoid sex or intimacy of other kinds. Phil had observed that most overweight women who had difficulty saying *no* to men also couldn't say *no* to their fathers. Many of these women are afraid that if they become too attractive they will get too many sexual advances from men and be unable to refuse them. So Phil recommended that women practice saying NO to men a lot, even about little things. I would also recommend the affirmation, "I can say *no* to people without losing their love."

These were some of the ideas we discussed the day I began this book. This conversation, and others with friends and clients, have helped me get clear on certain ideas many people have about weight and diet.

Many people are unhappy with their weight. They prefer to be thinner than they are, even if they are not greatly overweight. They try to make their bodies achieve an ideal weight or desired shape by punishing themselves in several ways. They deny their bodies food, imprisoning themselves in various restrictive diets or fasts, and force themselves to do exercises they do not enjoy. They keep on because they believe if they can change their bodies, their exteriors, they will be happier with themselves. They may lose weight and feel successful for a while, but eventually most of these people fail. Then they are even more unhappy with themselves.

These people have tried to start at the end by trying to change their physical bodies first. Your body cannot be separated from your self-image. To start at the beginning, you need to develop a complete and positive concept of yourself. You need to be at peace with yourself, to like yourself and others, and to treat yourself with love, not punishment. Your physical being does not take its shape directly from what you do to it, that is, from what you eat or how you exercise. Rather, your physical self responds to the attitude you have of it. Once your self-image improves, you can begin to reduce the inner strain and free your body of its outer fat. Your body is at the effect of your mind or, in other words, your mind always rules your body.

This book will show you how, by changing your thinking and your attitudes, you can change your weight and appearance. You can learn to love the self you are, and in loving that self, to become the self you want to be!

Introduction

You may have several reasons for wanting to lose weight. You may want to be thinner to attract or please a lover or just because you believe you would look better. Maybe you have added some inches as you have added some years. Not surprisingly, you associate gaining this weight with aging. You can't stop the calendar, but you can stop the scales!

You may feel that extra weight shows lack of discipline and enlightenment. Fat people are often considered to be unable to control their desires and their flabby bodies are supposed to prove it. Surely, you tell yourself, this is not me!

There are also health hazards to being overweight. If you are into science, the facts are that being even fifteen pounds over your average or best weight can reduce your life expectancy by as much as four years. Other scientific authorities have stated that being just ten pounds overweight carries a greater health risk than smoking twenty cigarettes a day.

Because being overweight, or merely thinking you are overweight, is so common in our society, a lot has been said and written about it. According to Dr. Hamburger, a psychologist, most eating disorders are symptomatic of depression, loneliness, boredom, sorrow, helplessness, guilt, and self-hate. One feeling leads to another and another in a circle you can't seem to break free of. "I eat because I'm depressed. I get depressed when I'm lonely. It's boring to be alone. . . " Do these feelings sound familiar to you?

Overweight people often have a sense of failure about being able to change their condition. They may become slaves to one diet after another. *This is a conspiracy against yourself!*

Along with diets, people often torture themselves physically in other ways. Jim Fadiman, a psychologist, says that any exercise done solely to lose weight won't do it in the long run. If you aren't exercising for pleasure, it is self-torture and just doing it reminds you that you are fat.

Our research through Rebirthing, which led to the Loving Relationships Training, has shown that overweight is also due to the birth trauma, parental disapproval syndrome, the unconscious death urge, and negative thought patterns. These four concepts are important to an understanding of the weight problem.

The *birth trauma* is your introduction to the world, to life outside the womb. Before birth you were in an ideal environment where all your needs were met—love, warmth, shelter, food. For most people being born is a violent experience that includes considerable pain and sense of loss. As a result of this experience, many people feel the world is a hostile, unpleasant place where untrustworthy people are out to get them. They may go through life apologizing for being born, seeking to return to the womb. This book will help you see the connection between the birth trauma and overeating.

The *parental disapproval syndrome* further sets you up for negative thinking about yourself and life. Your parents received disapproval when they were little, grew up, and passed disapproval on to you. This syndrome results from your parents failing to meet the demands of *their* parents for love and perfection. Your parents constantly failed to please their parents, who were demanding, and who withheld love and affection from them. As a result your parents spent a lot of time either trying to get back at their parents for the disapproval or trying to win their love. When these efforts failed, they suppressed their bitterness about it or transferred some of their resentment to other authority figures, such as teachers, mates, or employers.

After you were born, your parents could put on you the hostility they had inherited and lived with for so long This book will show you how your overeating is related to the parental disapproval syndrome.

The *unconscious death urge* is the acceptance of the inevitability of death by forces "out there." People accept the power of death when they refuse to question it. Many scientists are reporting spontaneous remissions and even cures from terminal illnesses, especially cancer, by patients who refuse to say *yes* to death. How many so-called miraculous cures have occurred through the centuries by people who refused to say *yes* to death can never accurately be determined. Many scientists are now admitting that the mind and its power over death must not be underestimated. Some scientists are now studying the spiritual masters and affirming what they have been preaching for centuries: There is an alternative to physical death and that is life extension/immortality, even the ability to dematerialize and rematerialize! Later in this book you will see the connection between overeating and the unconscious death urge.

Jesus Christ, recognized as a great spiritual teacher by non-Christian as well as Christian thinkers, said, "He who eats of my body shall live forever." Christianity, along with other religious thought, sees the sharing of food as symbolic of a deeper, more spiritual, mingling of souls. Breaking bread with others is truly a sacrament. But abusing food by overeating is a form of suicide and an unspoken death wish.

Negative thought patterns are all the negative thoughts

27

you love to beat yourself with regularly. They may include such favorites as "I never look right," "I can't ever have a good body," and "Nobody can ever love me because I'm too fat." To begin to change your pattern of weight tyranny, you must begin to change your thinking. You must learn to turn all your negative thoughts into positives in order to replace failure with success. You do not have to be stuck in futility and hopelessness. Being overweight is not natural unless you believe it is. *Anything you create with your mind you can uncreate.* You must uncreate the "heavy thoughts" that made you heavy.

Most people who are overweight have a life history of being overweight. They are overweight for a variety of reasons, and usually for more than one reason. From time to time they experience severe self-disgust or shame and decide to DO SOMETHING about it. So they diet and they exercise and they tune into various supposed weight-loss authorities. For a time they lose some pounds and feel successful. They like themselves and those around them. Then the pounds and the old fat silhouette return. This pattern happens over and over again. If you are one of these people, is it any surprise you feel the effort is futile and your case is hopeless?

The reason diet and other self-punishments have not worked for you and many other people is that you have never gotten to the *cause* of your weight problem. After a diet is over, your weight will come right back on if it is being used as protection for yourself or a weapon against someone else. This use comes from some fear that you must first uncover and then deal with. When the fear is gone, through the use of affirmations, Rebirthing, Rolfing, seminars or whatever works, you will be able to let the weight drop off naturally.

Let's start off by looking at the weight problem in another way. Here are some general points to ponder from the *Psychologist's Eat-Anything Diet* by Dr. Leonard Pearson:

Permanent weight loss takes place in an atmosphere of freedom.

Chronic dieters are in jail when they diet and are imprisoned by diet dictators.

Calorie counting perpetuates a state of futile warfare with yourself.

A common cause of overweight is not eating enough of what you love and crave.

Have you been losing the same twenty pounds for two decades? If you have the syndrome of dieting, losing some weight, panicking, gaining it back, going into self-pity, dieting again, etc., you demonstrate how inadequate and how incompetent you are and then your guilt will bring on more weight.

Do you have a syndrome of Person *vs* Food?

Do you eat through a filter of guilt?

I highly recommend this book by Pearson, which tells how you can get out of the tyranny you have put yourself into. It can help you start rethinking your approach to the whole weight problem.

Now here are some positive, not punishing, ways to start thinking about food and eating:

Eat the foods that "hum" to you.

Foods that hum to you are the ones that satisfy a particular hunger at a particular time.

Guilt and enjoyment make poor bedfellows.

Eating must give satisfaction and pleasure or it is ineffective.

The freedom to eat will also give you the freedom not to eat.

The Only Diet There Is is about a different kind of diet, a diet that can be done in bed. In fact, I highly recommend that you do do it in bed! This diet does NOT require you to give up food or do physical exercises. It DOES require you to diet from negative thinking and to do mental exercises. This diet can help you change your thinking, your feelings, and your appearance. It can make you feel good about yourself and your life. And isn't that what we all want?

Part One

About
The Only Diet There Is

The only diet there is is dieting from negative thinking. It is a diet of forgiveness and love!

If you love yourself and if you love your body and if you love food, this diet will always work. It is very inexpensive and it is very easy because all you have to do is lie in bed and follow the steps.

It is the last word on dieting because love is the highest thing there is and God is love and God is the highest thing there is.

Principles to Master First

1. Thought is creative and thoughts produce results. Positive thoughts produce for you positive results. Negative thoughts produce for you negative results. It is that simple.
2. It is not what you eat that can hurt you. It is what you BELIEVE about what you eat that can hurt you.
3. Therefore food is not "fattening" by itself. The thoughts you have about food are what make it fattening.
    a. A study done on people weighing precisely their desired weight showed that all of them could eat anything they wanted without any concern or worry.
    b. They could do so because all of them had one thing in common. They all had the thought that they could eat whatever and whenever they wanted without gaining weight. "I never gain weight" is simple enough.
4. Actually, our true nourishment comes to us from the light of God, not from food.
5. Any physical technique, such as fasting or special diets, works because your mind believes it will work. Unfortunately, until you handle the CAUSE of your overweight, you will most likely gain the weight back.

6. Your body always obeys the instructions of your mind. It is the instructions you give your body about food that matter.
7. Attitude and belief are the common denominators of all the causes of obesity.
   a. What causes you to be overweight is what you believe.
   b. The cause that never fails to produce results all the time is *thought*.
8. You must diet from negative thoughts about your body and food and yourself. That is *the only way to get* permanent results. To be successful, you must use positive thoughts.

Here are three important affirmations to try:

I, _____, *love myself.*
My body automatically processes whatever food I eat to maintain my perfect weight of _____, *pounds.*
Everything I eat turns to health and beauty.

If you have not used affirmations before, or if you have not been using them recently, read this section carefully. The key to positive thinking is the use of affirmations. Through the use of affirmations, you can program your mind and body for success.

An affirmation is a positive thought that you consciously choose to immerse in your consciousness to produce a certain desired result.

What you are doing is deliberately giving your mind an idea on which to act. Your mind will create what you want it to if you give it the opportunity. What you believe to be true, you create. Through repetition, you can program your mind to positive thoughts and thus achieve the goal you desire. You can use affirmations in several ways.

To begin with, write each affirmation ten or twenty times on a sheet of paper, leaving space at the right side for negative responses. As you write the affirmation on the left, write your negative responses or denials to it at the right. As you keep writing the affirmation, watch how your responses to it change. A stronger or key affirmation will bring up more negative responses from your unconscious, offering you the opportunity to see what stands between you and your goal.

When you can finally write the affirmation with only a neutral response, then and only then is your subconscious mind read to procede. These exercises will help you to become aware of what is already in your subconscious and where you are ready to go next.

After a week or so of writing an affirmation, or whenever your negative responses are quieted, you can stop using the response column and write only the affirmation. You may also want to use a tape cassette at this time, which I have found to be as effective, or to type your affirmations. I find typing allows me to write ten affirmations for each one I could otherwise write by hand.

You may want to say the affirmations to yourself. Although doing so takes less time, it is less powerful because it involves fewer senses than writing does.

Being able to write affirmations is important to success with this program. Try to enjoy finding out more about yourself as you use it.

EXAMPLES:

I, _____, deserve to maintain my perfect weight of 126 pounds.

I, _____, deserve to maintain my perfect weight of 126 pounds, no matter what I eat.

RESPONSES:

I don't believe it.

That would be too good to be true.

I, _____, deserve to maintain my perfect weight of 126 pounds, no matter what I eat.

I wouldn't know what to do if I were perfect; what would I worry about?

I, _____, deserve to maintain my perfect weight of 126 pounds, no matter what I eat.

Yes, it's a good idea but how?

It's easy for me to maintain my perfect weight of 126 pounds if I think so.

Ha!

Basic Steps to the Diet

Before you begin this diet, you must prepare yourself for it by being willing to "get off it." By getting off it, I mean being willing to give up your weight case now. Are you willing to give up all those payoffs, all those real and secret rewards you get from being overweight? Are you willing to give up getting attention or avoiding attention? Are you willing to experience out the fear your fat is hiding? Are you willing to give up your misery? Are you willing to let go of all that now and be free?

If you ask yourself "Am I willing to get off it now?" and the answer comes back "No," then even this ultimate diet won't work! You are not ready for it yet. You might even be sad about giving up something you are so attached to, even if it is neurotic!

The first step is always to tell the truth. You can start by asking yourself what payoffs you are getting now. That is, think about what you really get out of being fat, what do you get to prove? Here are some examples. You can make your own list.

What are my payoffs for being overweight?

EXAMPLES:

1. I get to prove that I am not perfect.
2. I get to prove that my mother is wrong.
3. I get to be angry at myself.
4. I get to punish myself.
5. I get to stay out of Heaven.
6. I get to keep too many men/women from wanting to make love to me.
7. I get to have a problem to get attention.
8. I get to feel helpless about this problem.
9. I get to have a reason for failing.
10. I get to complain.

The next part of preparing yourself is being willing to give up all those payoffs. Each one of them can be changed into an affirmation.

1. It is okay for me, _____, to be perfect.
2. I, _____, no longer need to get even with my mother and prove her wrong.
3. I, _____, forgive myself and therefore I am never angry at myself.
4. I, _____, refuse to punish myself ever again.
5. I, _____, am ready to stay in Heaven *now!*
6. It is okay to have lots of men/women wanting to make love to me. I can say no if I want to.
7. I, _____, do not need a problem to get attention.
8. I, _____, no longer feel helpless about this problem.
9. I, _____, am successful and so I no longer need an explanation for failing.
10. I, _____, have given up complaining.

If you are not willing to get off it now, then become willing to be willing. After you do the affirmations related to your payoff you will become willing soon.

My payoffs for being overweight are:

_____

_____

_____

_____

_____

_____

_____

_____

_____

_____

My new affirmations are:

_____

_____

_____

_____

_____

_____

_____

_____

_____

_____

_____

Step One: Diet from Negative Thinking

Here are some samples of negative thinking. Write your own thoughts in the column at the right.

Here are all my negative thoughts about my body and weight:

EXAMPLES:

1. I can't lose weight just by thinking about it.

1. _____

2. It is hard to lose weight.

2. _____

3. If I get fat, something terrible will happen to me.

3. _____

4. Watch out what you eat because you will get fat.

4. _____

5. It will never work. No diets work.

5. _____

6. I cannot get my body exactly right.

6. _____

7. This is taking too long.

7. _____

8. It is hopeless.

8. _____

9. Nothing works when it comes to losing weight.

9. _____

10. If I don't get this, then something is wrong with me. I am not enlightened.

10. _____

Here are all my negative thoughts about food:

1. I can't win when it comes to food.

1. _____
_____

2. Bread is fattening.

2. _____

3. Ice cream is fattening.

3. _____

4. The most pleasurable foods are dangerous.

4. _____
_____

5. You have to eat a certain amount of each nutrient or you will die.

5. _____
_____
_____

6. Food is the most important thing there is.

6. _____
_____

7. A woman should always prepare the food and serve it to a man.

7. _____
_____
_____

8. Food is dangerous.

8. _____

9. I give up because I hate food.

9. _____
_____

10. Food is first, then love.

10. _____

Step Two: Feast on Affirmations

The second step is to change your negative thoughts into affirmations. Diet from the negative and feed on the positive thoughts. Remember, these are the only exercises I promised you would have! Here are some sample affirmations. Write your responses at the right.

Here are all my affirmations about my body and weight:

EXAMPLES:

1. I, _____, can lose weight just by the power of my mind.

1. _____
   _____
   _____

2. It is easy for me, _____, to lose weight.

2. _____
   _____

3. Nothing terrible will happen to me, _____, no matter what I weigh.

3. _____
   _____
   _____

4. I, _____, am now eating my way to thinness.

4. _____
   _____

5. This diet always works.

5. _____

6. I, _____, can now get my body exactly right.

6. _____
   _____

7. This is taking the right amount of time.

7. _____
   _____

8. This is working now!

8. _____

9. I, _____, am fine no matter what happens.

9. _____
   _____

10. I, _____, can definitely resolve this problem.

10. _____
    _____

Here are all my affirmations about food:

EXAMPLES:

1. I, _____, always win with food.

2. Bread is not fattening. I, _____, can eat bread and be slim.

3. I, _____, can be slim and stay slim eating ice cream.

4. The most pleasurable foods are not fattening to me, _____. They are actually slimming.

5. I, _____, will not die whether I eat or not.

6. Food is not the most important thing to me, _____.

7. I, _____, do not have to prepare and serve food just because I am a woman. I, _____, can prepare and serve food even if I am a man.

8. Food is safe for me, _____.

9. I, _____, love food but I can take it or leave it.

10. Love is always first for me, _____, and then I don't need food to get love.

1. _____

_____

2. _____

_____

_____

3. _____

_____

_____

4. _____

_____

_____

_____

5. _____

_____

6. _____

_____

7. _____

_____

_____

_____

_____

8. _____

_____

9. _____

_____

10. _____

_____

_____

You will feel more comfortable with some affirmations than with others. Hence, they will work better for you. Here are the best general affirmations about diet.

My body processes everything I, _____, eat automatically to maintain my perfect weight of _____ pounds.

Everything I, _____, eat turns to health and beauty.

I, _____, deserve the pleasure I receive from eating.

I, _____, am losing weight and gaining beauty now.

I, _____, am pleasing to myself whether I eat or not. or not.

Infinite Intelligence within me, _____, always does the right thing to maintain my perfect weight of _____ pounds.

That which is pleasurable to me, _____, no longer has any undesirable consequences.

The more satisfaction I, _____, experience, the less emptiness I experience.

My life and health are really sustained by the Light of God.

All food I, _____, attract is good for me and I eat for pleasure. I do not attract food that would not be good for me.

My metabolism is responding to the new instructions that I, _____, am giving it.

I, _____, have the right to change my parents' rules about eating.

I, _____, am willing to see the truth about my weight problem.

I, _____, am okay whether I am thin or not.

I, _____, can get love whether I eat or not.

I, _____, can say "no" without losing others' love.

I, _____, am totally healed of this problem.

Calories have only the power that I, _____, give them.

My mind rules my body.

Do these general affirmations regularly.

1. Write the most significant ones at least ten times a day.
2. Paste them on a wall or mirror where you will see them.
3. Think them in meditations.
4. Say them to a friend sitting across from you and have the friend say "thank you" after each one.
5. Put them on a tape cassette in the first and third person and listen to them each night.

In addition, I recommend you read the chapter on weight in *Rebirthing in the New Age.** Listen to Leonard Orr's taped seminar about weight. These can be obtained by writing to Inspiration University, Box 234, Sierraville, California 96126.

**Rebirthing in the New Age* by Leonard Orr and Sondra Ray, published by Celestial Arts, Millbrae, California.

All my negative thoughts about my body are:

_____
_____
_____
_____
_____
_____
_____
_____

All my negative thoughts about my weight are:

_____
_____
_____
_____
_____
_____
_____
_____

All my negative thoughts about food are:

_____
_____
_____
_____
_____
_____
_____

My new affirmations about my body are:

_____
_____
_____
_____
_____
_____
_____
_____

My new affirmations about my weight are:

_____
_____
_____
_____
_____
_____
_____

My new affirmations about food are:

_____
_____
_____
_____
_____
_____
_____

Step Three: Use Visualizations

If you are able to visualize well when you close your eyes, take advantage of this ability and "see" yourself in your ideal form and shape, weighing your ideal weight. Lie or sit in meditation daily and visualize your body the way you want it to be. *What you think about expands.* If you are thinking about your body being fat, it will expand and you will get fatter. If you think about the ideal slim body you want, the slimness will expand and you will get more of that!

If you are not able to visualize well, put up a photograph of yourself taken when you were your ideal weight and when you were happy. Look at it a few quiet moments each day. If you do not have a photo, use a magazine picture of someone with a body like the one you want. You can paste a photo of your face over the other person's. Look at the picture every day.

Don't be jealous when you see someone who looks just the way you want to look. Instead of resenting that person, say, "That's for me!"

You can change not only your weight this way. You can also change your features, contours, and over-all appearance.

Step Four: Give up Anger

Before you can give up your anger, which is the next step, ask yourself the following question: "Who do I get to blame by keeping this problem?" That person's name has already appeared in your consciousness. That person MUST be forgiven.

A *Course in Miracles* explains that all distress is due to unforgiveness and that forgiveness is our only function. Forgiveness is also the Master Erase. Forgiveness means forgiving yourself and forgiving others as well. It means getting clear on what you are angry about and then letting go of it. Forgiveness is selective remembering. It is remembering only the loving thoughts you received and gave. All else must be forgotten. Forgive and you will see things differently. Forgive and the problem will disappear.

You can start to give up your anger by asking this question. Then answer it truthfully for yourself.

What am I angry about?
1.   I am angry at my father for _____.
2.   I am angry at my mother for _____.
3.   I am angry at myself for being so _____.
4.   I am angry at women for _____.
5.   I am angry at men for _____.
6.   I am angry at myself for failing to _____.

Now go on with the following statements about yourself. Some of the answers may be similar.

What have I not forgiven myself for yet?
1.   I have not forgiven myself for _____.
2.   Another thing I have not forgiven myself for is_____

    _____.
3.   I have not forgiven myself for eating _____.
4.   I have not forgiven myself for being _____.
5.   I have not forgiven myself for thinking _____

    _____.
6.   I have not forgiven myself for saying _____.
7.   I have not forgiven myself for acting _____.

8. I have not forgiven myself for blaming others about ___

9. I have not forgiven myself for hurting _____.
10. I have not forgiven myself for not giving _____

_____.

What have I not forgiven others for yet?
1. I have not forgiven my father for _____.
2. I have not forgiven my mother for _____.
3. I have not forgiven my brother/sister for _____

_____.
4. I have not forgiven my lover for _____.
5. I have not forgiven _____ for hurting me.
6. I have not forgiven _____ for not speaking to me.
7. I have not forgiven _____ for refusing to loan me money.
8. I have not forgiven _____ for lying to me.
9. I have not forgiven _____ for saying things about me.
10. I have not forgiven _____ for leaving me.

All these people should be forgiven, whether you like it or not!

Begin now to give up your anger by forgiving yourself and others. Rewrite each statement to make it fit you.

1. I forgive myself for _____.
2. Another thing I forgive myself for is _____.
3. I forgive myself for eating _____.
4. I forgive myself for being _____.
5. I forgive myself for thinking _____.
6. I forgive myself for saying _____.
7. I forgive myself for acting _____.

8. I forgive myself for blaming others about _____ .
9. I forgive myself for hurting _____ .
10. I forgive myself for not giving _____ .

1. I forgive my father for _____ .
2. I forgive my mother for _____ .
3. I forgive my brother/sister for _____ .
4. I forgive my lover for _____ .
5. I forgive _____ for hurting me.
6. I forgive _____ for not speaking to me.
7. I forgive _____ for refusing to loan me money.
8. I forgive _____ for lying to me.
9. I forgive _____ for saying things to me.
10. I forgive _____ for leaving me.

In the name of Jesus, all is forgiven. I ask the Holy Spirit for a correction of all my wrong thinking now!

Here are five steps to complete forgiveness, from Catherine Ponder. Think about them!

1. You forgive others.
2. They forgive you.
3. You forgive yourself.
4. You give up all claim to punishment.
5. You restore harmony as it was before the event.

Most people work out their anger on other people in violent and harmful ways. There are more socially acceptable and even loving ways to cleanse yourself of anger. You can go off by yourself in your car, in the garage or some other solitary place, and scream. You can go outside by yourself to the woods, a beach, or some secluded place and scream. If you prefer to stay indoors, you can pound on pillows. Or you can lie in bed (I said this whole process could be done in bed!)

and start kicking your legs up and down, higher and higher, keeping your knees straight, until you get it all out. You can also use boffing sticks and work off your anger in a mock fight with someone else.

All these ways to clean out anger feel wonderful. Do whichever one or ones work for you, but do them daily. Be sure you breathe during any of these activities. Don't be surprised if you feel like crying afterwards. This is very good! Also, scream your affirmations!

You express your anger in order to drop it. Don't hang on to it. You can work it out in five minutes or you can drag it out for five hours. It's better to give it up!

Step Five: Write Down Your Feelings

During this process it is a good idea to keep a notebook of all your feelings, especially when you feel upset. You will learn a great deal about yourself this way. You will begin to see patterns in why you act and feel as you do. You will begin to understand yourself and to choose other ways to solve your problems.

The best time to write is when you feel like eating, even though you are not really hungry. Instead of eating, next time take out a notebook and begin to write down your feelings. Write how you really feel. Remember, you are writing only to yourself about yourself.

Later, read your entries. Then write weight affirmations and other affirmations that apply to what you wrote. Then, and only then, eat if you still want to. Chances are, you won't feel like it any more.

Here is a sample notebook entry.

Tuesday night. I want to eat bread! Lots and lots of bread! I want to eat bread because I am angry. My grandmother was angry a lot and she baked a lot of bread. Am I being my grandmother??? Yes! I am taking care of everything and everybody like she did. Am I ever going to be free?

I have no discipline at all! I am angry at myself for having no discipline. That is not really true! I have had discipline before. I don't have it now because I want to be angry. Beating myself up for breaking a fast is a good way to stay angry at myself. Maybe I even go on fasts just so I can break them! No, that really is ridiculous! Or is it? What can I do?

I can either:
1. Fast and be disciplined. (This won't work.)
2. Fast, break the fast, and forgive myself. (This hasn't worked.)
3. Forgive myself first and then eat. (I don't want to do this.)
4. Forgive myself first and then fast. (I don't know.)

What do I REALLY want? To eat or not eat and to feel good either way. Now I eat the things I most forbid myself to eat (bread, butter, and ice cream) so I can get most angry at myself.

What I am really angry at is men! (God is a man!) I just got a pain in my side. It all seems hopeless. I feel like an alcoholic. I don't want to give up but I am *fed up.* Can I ever get over this?

Sometime after this first writing session, you might go on to think through your anger. Here is a later entry.

I am not my grandmother. I don't have to be angry just because she was. I don't have to eat bread and butter, but if I choose to anyway, I can create them not to be fattening. Either way is okay.

I am not helpless. I do have discipline. I am disciplining myself right now to handle this. I do not have to fast in order to handle this. I am handling this right now. I no longer must go on fasts just to break them and get angry at myself. I no longer get angry at myself. I refuse to punish myself ever again. I am fine whether I eat or I don't eat. I approve of myself all the time now.

I forgive all men. I forgive myself for thinking God did something to me. God is just waiting to help me with this and now I can let Him.

Another way to write down your feelings is to send yourself a letter. Who else knows better how much you deserve a little recognition? Tell yourself on paper about the progress you know you are making and then mail the letter.

Dear Sondra,

I am happy to see that you are really getting off it. I see that you are looking younger and more beautiful and that you have lost weight. Are you ever looking great! I think you should certainly acknowledge yourself for getting your thoughts under control and working out those fears that made you put on weight. You will never have to go through this again because you got down to the CAUSE. I really am proud of you! You deserve to be rewarded so I am treating you to a massage! You deserve to be your ideal weight of 126 pounds.

Love,

a friend

Step Six: Bless Your Food

When you eat, *love* your food and it will love you back. Begin by blessing the food. Food is a form of energy that cannot harm you or do something to you if you do not want it to. Say, "This food I eat only turns to health and beauty."

Enjoy the beauty of your food. Clean other things unrelated to eating, such as school work or newspapers, off the table. When you serve food, don't slop it on the table any which way. Use enough plates or bowls for serving so that each kind of food is made more attractive. That way you can see the health and beauty you are about to consume.

Make your mealtimes more spiritual. Whether you eat alone or with others, enjoy your food. Enjoy talking with others or rethinking a pleasant happening of the day. Don't eat while you are reading or watching television and ignore the food. Look at the food you are eating, experience its smell and taste, and think about what you are doing. Take time to relax when you eat and savor each bite. Take a deep breath each time you put something into your mouth.

Step Seven: Love Your Body

If you love your body, it will cooperate with your mind. Develop a loving relationbship with your body. Treat it the way you would treat your dearest friend. If you have been saying that your body does not cooperate with you, then your perfect weight can never be achieved. You are in a continuous state of noncooperation with your body. If you say "I don't like my body," then your body must do whatever you DON'T want it to do in order to please you! (GET THAT!) As a result, your body will go on getting heavier and heavier.

You should love your body even if it is overweight because it is doing what you want. On some level, you want to be overweight so your body is giving you what you secretly want. Your body is always obedient to your mind. If you are telling your body to lose weight and it is *not* doing that, you must have a deeper COUNTER INTENTION that your mind is putting out. Check this out with yourself.

If you think you may be in a state of noncooperation with yourself, analyze your responses to this next affirmation until you find out the counter intention.

AFFIRMATION:

I, _____, am willing to lose weight now.

RESPONSES:

Not yet because I'd be perfect.

It's not safe to be thin.

Step Eight: Pleasure Yourself

It is very important that you pleasure yourself while you are going on this diet! This is a diet of love. You must love your body, love the food you eat, and love those you are angry at. But most of all, you must love yourself in every way. Therefore it is important that you give yourself some deep, sensuous pleasures. A frequent, even daily massage, for example, would be ideal.

Never say to yourself that you cannot afford some special pleasure, such as a massage. If you can get that a massage is about receiving, and that your financial status is also related to receiving, you will see that the more you receive pleasure during a massage, the more you will open yourself to receiving in every way, including money. So massages can definitely increase your prosperity! You may even get a multi-million dollar idea on the massage table! But most important to get is that a massage is also a way of loving your body.

Another way to pleasure yourself is to take a luxurious bath. I recommend soaking twice a day. Take the time to get the water temperature exactly right. Get something to read or music to listen to, if you want, and plenty of soft towels. This is a great way to love yourself and also to meditate.

You should do anything at all that brings you pleasure during this period. Most people are hard on themselves while they are on a diet. Remember this is not a diet of denial. You do not even deny yourself food! This is a diet of love and it would be a good idea for you to get in touch with whatever gives you pleasure and how you want to be loved. You can start to figure this out by making a pleasures list.

You have five senses, five key ways to receive pleasure: by seeing, smelling, tasting, touching, and hearing. Try to include something for each one in your list. You may get pleasure in other ways too, perhaps from remembering or imagining.

Here are my ten greatest pleasures:

1. <u>I love to soak for hours in soothing warm water.</u>
2. _____
3. _____
4. _____
5. _____
6. _____
7. _____
8. _____
9. _____
10. _____

After you have made out your list of pleasures, think about how these pleasures relate to ways to receive love from yourself and others. Now translate your pleasures into specific ways of loving and being loved.

Ten ways I could love myself are:

1. <u>I will start to use a hot tub at least once a week.</u>
2. _____
3. _____
4. _____
5. _____
6. _____
7. _____
8. _____
9. _____
10. _____

Ten ways I could let others love me are:

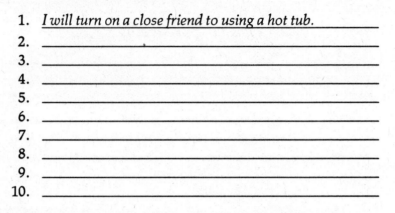

1. *I will turn on a close friend to using a hot tub.*
2. _____
3. _____
4. _____
5. _____
6. _____
7. _____
8. _____
9. _____
10. _____

The more love you give and receive, the more energy will be unblocked in your body.

Step Nine: Turn It All Over to God

Ask God for a correction in your thinking about all these matters. Ask for help in releasing all your negative thoughts about food and weight. Be willing to receive assistance. Every time you catch yourself indulging in negative thoughts like, "It is hopeless," "This won't work," "I can never lose weight," invert these thoughts to affirmations. If you seem unable to get unstuck from them, merely say "I give this to God" or "I turn this over to the Holy Spirit" or "I allow the Holy Spirit to undo all my wrong thinking about my body, food and weight."

You can also use the mantra OM NAMA SHIVAYA, which is the ultimate mantra. It means "Oh Lord Shiva, I bow before thee in reverence," which translates one way to mean "I surrender to that part of God that destroys ignorance." Shiva is the destroyer of ignorance. In this way you can destroy those ignorant thoughts that cause you to gain weight. It also means "Infinite Spirit, Infinite Being and Infinite Manifestation."

Ernest Holmes created a method called the "Golden Key." He suggested that when you are stuck, stop thinking about the problem and start thinking about God. If you cannot grasp how to think about God, think of the words *peace*, *harmony*, *bliss*, *joy*, and anything that produces these results for you! God is _____.

Pray for the removal of the fear of giving up this problem. After all, you probably would have given it up easily by now if you did not have some fear of doing so.

Be aware of the dynamics of miracles, from the children's material in *A Course in Miracles*.

1. Recognize that a healing must take place. (Losing weight is a healing, if that is your desired result.)
2. Then ask the Holy Spirit for guidance.
3. Listen to the answer you will receive.
4. Faithfully trust in the sure guidance of the Holy Spirit.

Step Ten: Give Thanks

Give thanks to God that the problem is already resolved. Come from certainty and faith. Love and relaxation give you power. You have the power to handle this and other problems. Now your higher self wants to acknowledge that ability and to offer thanks for it. Doing this will always bring fast results! Always!

Write your ideal weight on a piece of paper and tape it to the mirror.

Don't
   eat
      when
        you
         are
           upset!

Think
    thin
        24 hours
      a
        day!

Part Two

Getting Started

Here again are the steps for *The Only Diet There Is:*

1. Diet from negative thinking.
2. Feast on affirmations.
3. Use visualizations.
4. Give up anger.
5. Write down your feelings.
6. Bless your food.
7. Love your body.
8. Pleasure yourself.
9. Turn it all over to God.
10. Give thanks to God.

I can't give you a calendar or a timetable for how long you will need to work your way through these ten steps. Only your body knows how long it took you to get in the mental and physical condition you are in now. You must get reacquainted with your body and work out your problems with it.

It took me six to eight months to get clear on Part Two of this book. It came to me as a result of praying for mastery and the research I did on myself and my clients and students. This part of the book will help you with specific blocks you may have in working through the ten steps of the diet.

Because much of your problem with your body has to do with problems in your thinking, that is where this diet begins and keeps returning. To help your body to change, you must first change your thinking. That change can best take place through using affirmations. For that reason, each chapter ends with some affirmations to help you overcome specific mental blocks. Do the affirmations as you need to, according to the suggested plan at the beginning of the Principles chapter. Use your name in the affirmations each time you write or say them. Address yourself in the first, second, and third persons this way:

"I, _Sondra_, can be successful with _The Only Diet There Is_."
"You, _Sondra_, can be successful with _The Only Diet There Is_."
"She, _Sondra_, can be successful with _The Only Diet There Is_."

Use an affirmation in all three forms because your thinking has been conditioned in these ways from your conscious mind and from messages you received from others. Remember to involve as many senses as you can by writing, saying, reading, and listening to the affirmations that can most help you.

I Deserve to Be
My Ideal Weight

I, _____, *deserve to be my ideal weight.*

When I tried other affirmations, such as "I am losing weight now" or "I can stay on a diet," they never worked because I had too big a charge on the words *lose* and *diet*. But the words *ideal weight* were pleasant enough to me that this affirmation worked superbly.

I put *deserve* in the affirmation because I wanted to get that I was good enough to have what I wanted. I was good enough to look great and receive compliments about my body. I was good enough to get the pleasure of wearing beautiful clothes. I was good enough to let myself get over my neuroses about worrying about my weight.

In other words, I had to convince myself that I deserved to be happy. I was a child of God and I loved myself. Jesus said, Love thy neighbor AS THYSELF. To love your neighbor, you must first experience what love is by loving yourself.

The degree to which you think you don't deserve to be your ideal weight is the degree to which you still hate yourself. One reason people hate themselves is because they see themselves as separate from God. Seeing yourself apart from God puts you in a position of isolation and total helplessness. You end up saying things like "I can't lose weight" or "I can't lose weight without dieting." Any sentence with "I can't" in it immediately puts you into total helplessness. Obviously what works is "I can, with the help of God, easily be my ideal weight."

I always try to see myself as part of God, as a cell in God's body. Therefore I have all the power of God, the source, to help me clear up anything. The truth is that I am already perfect and clear and complete in God, and whenever I don't think so, the thought is something I made up and an illusion. Therefore when I was overweight, it was something I had made up because I was afraid.

Affirmations About My Ideal Weight:

1. I, _____, deserve to have a fantastic body.
2. I, _____, deserve to look great in whatever I choose to wear.
3. I, _____, deserve to get compliments on how great I look.
4. I, _____, deserve to be happy.
5. Because I, _____, am a child of God, I love myself.
6. I, _____, am perfect and complete now because I am a part of God.
7. As part of God, I, _____, am also part of the Divine Source of power.
8. I, _____, have the power to succeed with whatever I choose to do.
9. With the help of God, I, _____, can easily be my ideal weight.
10. I, _____, deserve to be my ideal weight.

Retained Hate Is Overweight

Love is fluid, moving, and light. Hate is heavy, thick, and dark. Chances are that your excess weight, which is just stuck energy, is the extra hate you are carrying around. All conditions that are not in the ideal form come from nonforgiveness, as you can see in *A Course In Miracles*. If being overweight is something you want to change, then it is not an ideal condition. Therefore you must ask yourself, "Who do I get to blame by hanging on to this overweight?" Let the truth surface. "Who am I hating?" That person has to be forgiven.

Overweight is also a reflection of one's own self-hate. What are you hating yourself for? You can make a list of times when you were ashamed, even angry at yourself. Then you must begin to forget these things and forgive yourself. Change your criticism into praise and affirmations. If you are used to having that hate for yourself or someone else, just saying "I forgive him/her" or "I forgive myself" may not be enough. You must use affirmations continuously, repeating them until forgiveness is total.

You will know when you have totally forgiven by the result you get. Results are your guru. When you become your ideal weight, you have forgiven. It is good to say in a prayer "I am ready to forgive now, help me." That means you are ready to give up all resentment and blame of yourself and others.

I have found that most people want to forgive the hate and anger of their past, all those things they think were "done to them," but they can't. Either they do not know how to forgive or they are afraid to do so. These feelings have become so much a part of their lives they are a kind of habit.

These people also have a habit of blaming others. As long as you are blaming others for anything that happens to you, you will not be able to clear it up or get the lesson that the universe is trying to teach you. Then it will come around again with more intensity. You might even get fatter until you get so "fed up" you are finally FORCED to look at the truth.

If you ask for results and help with forgiveness but you feel you do not get it, don't blame God. You aren't really ready, that's all. You probably have too much fear. The Holy Spirit will never add to your fear. Actually, you should pray for the release of the FEAR of giving up being overweight, instead of praying directly to lose weight. Your desires to lose weight may be blocked by various fears.

You may fear giving up the overweight because you are using it for protection. If you didn't have it, you might feel "too good" and "too good" might somehow be dangerous. People often have it wired up that it is bad to feel too good. They actually fear happiness. For them, misery seems a more natural condition.

You may also fear giving up overweight because then other people would be too interested in you sexually. If people got too interested in you in this way, you might have a lot of sexual offers and that is somehow "bad" or "frightening." You may fear giving up overweight because without the burden of those extra pounds you would feel too light and too high. You don't really believe those good feelings will last because you fear someone or something will bring you "down." Somehow, you think, it is safer to bring yourself down first. Having something to worry about seems safer. If I get too high or too perfect, something bad might happen to me, the ego will insist.

The moral of this story is that it is SAFE to give up hate, safe to stop blaming others, and safe to stop fearing your own good feelings. People intuitively know that if they give up hate and forgive everything they would have a lot more energy. A lot more. They would have a lot more of God. If someone is afraid of the energy, which is God, then he or she won't want more and will try to avoid getting more by staying in hate. This is important to get.

It is also important to realize that more energy is not dangerous and God is not dangerous because God does not kill people. People kill themselves and therefore all death is suicide. Once again, when you get what God is, you aren't afraid to have more. Because God is energy added to our thoughts, all our thoughts get more and more powerful the longer we live. Suppressed hate thoughts will thus also get more energy added to them, and as the overweight increases, the pain gets greater.

Affirmations About Hate and Forgiveness:

1. I, _____, am ready to stop being afraid of feeling too good.
2. I, _____, am ready to give up being afraid that other people may be sexually attracted to me.
3. I, _____, am ready to accept feeling light and happy as my natural state.
4. It is now safe for me, _____, to feel good about myself all the time.
5. It is safe for me, _____, to totally forgive everyone in my past and present.

6. It is safe for me, _____, to give up all fear and hate.
7. I, _____, am ready to forgive myself because I am overweight.
8. I, _____, am ready to forgive others and stop blaming them, especially _____, for my overweight.
9. I, _____, am ready to give up resenting and blaming myself for my overweight.
10. I, _____, am ready to forgive it all now, God. Please help me.

It Is Safe to Be Happy

One day I realized that I was very unhappy about constantly worrying over food and overweight, two things which seemed to plague me continuously. Since we think about food so many times a day, I had many, many opportunities to be unhappy. I wondered why I was repeatedly choosing to be unhappy by constantly worrying about food or my body. Why didn't I just choose to stop worrying and be happy? Then I realized I was afraid to be completely happy because it seemed the times when I was the happiest were followed by something terrible. Somehow it was better to stay in a state of slight unhappiness rather than soar high and then crash.

Only the ego could make up such insanity! When I realized that I had tricked myself into staying unhappy by using worries about food and my body, I realized I did so because of fear. But fear is a function of the ego, that is, fear is something I made up and was doing to myself. Then I realized I do not have to hold onto fear, to stay slightly unhappy, or to worry that something terrible would happen if I became "too happy." All I had to get is that I am safe and Immortal right now if I say so. It is also safe for me to be happy. *A Course in Miracles* says "God's will for me is perfect happiness."

However, before you can accept your birthright of happiness, you must give up GUILT. Guilt also makes you heavy. Guilt, like hate, is a cover for fear. As *A Course in Miracles* explains, both hate and guilt come under the category of fear You are either into the ego, which is fear, or God, who is love. Therefore if you are guilty whenever you eat something, you are into the ego. If you are saying to yourself, "I should not eat this," you are into guilt and fear and punishment of yourself. Of course you will gain weight, and probably on that very mouthful!

If you are saying "I love myself for eating this," then the energy will flow and you will transmute the food into love and energy and it will not get stuck as fat. However, if you are using your fat to keep away sex or whatever, you will not allow yourself to stop saying "I shouldn't eat this" because your payoff is too great.

You have worked out for yourself a whole trip of "beating yourself up" by getting overweight, dieting in pain, worrying about gaining it all back, and hating yourself every time you eat. In order to let go of this trip, you have to be totally willing to give up the ENTIRE syndrome, which includes the payoffs you are now getting out of it. Therefore I suggest you do a little truth process with yourself. It requires three pieces of paper, a pen or pencil, and a willingness to be totally honest with yourself.

At the top of the first page, write the following sentence and then add your own reasons:

I have this extra weight for the following reasons:

1. *I don't like myself.* _____
2. _____
3. _____
4. _____
5. _____

On page two, list the real payoffs you are getting out of your overweight problem.

The payoffs I get out of having this extra weight are:

1. *I prove I'm not good enough.* _____
2. _____
3. _____
4. _____
5. _____

Then on page three, write the reasons why you are afraid to change.

The fears I have of letting go of this problem are:

1. *I'd be too good without it.* _____
2. _____
3. _____
4. _____
5. _____

When you have told the TOTAL truth, you will probably have a bunch of negative thoughts on your three lists. Invert them into personal affirmations for yourself. From the first list, for example:

My biggest payoff for staying fat is that I get to prove I am ugly and nobody likes me.

Change that into this affirmation:

I, _____, am now willing for my beauty to come out and I am now willing for everyone to like me.

This affirmation is perhaps the best:

Because I, _____, am one with God, it is safe for me to be my ideal weight.

Always remember that God is love and love is the only safety there is.

Affirmations About Safety and Happiness:

1. I, _____, can eat anything I want without feeling guilty or unhappy.
2. I, _____, feel safe and happy when I eat.
3. I, _____, love myself for eating whatever makes me happy.
4. I, _____, feel safe and have no fear of any foods I eat.
5. I, _____, feel safe and have no fear of giving up my overweight problem.
6. I, _____, am willing to like myself and be happy now.
7. It is safe for me, _____, to let others get close to me and like me.
8. I, _____, am now willing to let my natural good looks show.
9. I, _____, am willing for others to see how attractive I am.
10. Because I, _____, am one with God, it is safe for me to be my ideal weight.

Pleasure Yourself to Thinness

If thinness is your goal, then more pleasure will get you there faster. But what most people do is to avoid pleasure and punish themselves for being overweight, which just adds more pounds. (Heavy thoughts can make you "heavy.") The more these people beat themselves up with such thoughts as "You shouldn't have!" "How stupid you are for eating that!" and "Aren't you terrible looking!" the more they hate themselves, the more nervous they get, and the more they eat. If they still believe food is fattening, of course they will get even fatter

Are you one of these people? Do you say to yourself, "There is no end to this trap of misery"?

Now, try a whole new system!

Focus on pleasure. Do whatever you know gives pleasure to yourself and makes you happy. Then you will be loving yourself. Remember that love is fluid and moving. If you are happy, your molecules will start moving and your extra weight, or stuck molecules, will move around. Get massaged, have more sex, go to a sauna, treat yourself—you know what is best!

You will have a tendency NOT to do the things that give you pleasure while you are hating your body for not being what you think it should be. If you do not break this chain and start doing good things to your body, you will sink into more hate and get stuck. No diet will work for you then. You will only gain back the weight soon since you never totally stopped hating yourself.

The answer then is more pleasure, more love. Therefore it follows that eating the things that please you is wiser than painful dieting. If you deny yourself eating foods that please you, you are hating yourself by denying yourself what you want. This denial is very subtle but your mind knows when you are ripping yourself off. Then you feel cheated and angry. Anger, which caused your overweight to begin with, is heavy and it will increase and get you even more stuck.

Affirmations About Pleasure:

1. I, _____, love myself and I want to give love and pleasure to myself.
2. I, _____, deserve all the love and pleasure I can give myself.
3. Because I, _____, eat for pleasure, I do not gain weight from food.
4. Because I, _____, love myself, I feel happy and light.
5. As I get more pleasure daily, I, _____, am also getting thinner.
6. Because I am getting thinner, I, _____, deserve even more pleasure.
7. My body knows what foods will give me the most pleasure.
8. My body wants to eat only those foods that are safe and pleasing to me.
9. I, _____, love my body as it is now.
10. Because I, _____, love my body, I want to give it more pleasure each day.

Eating By Yourself

While you are working through this process, it is a good idea to take one meal a day alone and in silence to experience the food totally. My friend Jim Morningstar had this suggestion, which proved very valuable to me.

If, as a child, your meals at home had a lot of tension and suppressed hate or fear or outright disapproval, eating with others may not have been very pleasant. Perhaps you couldn't wait to get away from the table, especially if meals were when you got all the bad news in your family. Therefore you probably did not get to experience the total *pleasure* of food. Or maybe you were so busy talking or trying to be heard over the others at the table that you never let yourself stop long enough to taste what was in your mouth. Now, as an adult, you may never have felt truly nourished by food or allowed yourself to be totally pleasured by it. You are still walking away from the table, still feeling ripped off.

Eating alone can help you take your time, unbothered by anyone or anything, to experience the real enjoyment of eating. When you finally experience the pleasure of food you will not have to eat so much (for those who still believe food is fattening). Or else you will be so pleasured that you will let yourself eat a great deal (for those who have integrated the thought that food is not fattening but only obeys your instructions).

I once met a Rolfer named Barry who usually ate by himself. He set the table with fine china to make each meal an occasion, and ate by candlelight. I was very impressed with his love for himself. He obviously knew the difference between being lonely and being alone. You feel lonely when you feel deprived of the company of others or rejected by them. But when you choose to be alone, you have the opportunity to enjoy your own company and appreciate your self-worth. Get into the joy of solitude.

Some poeple who have their meals alone would rather eat standing up than face a table with nobody sitting across from them. These are the people who say, "Oh, that's too much trouble to fix just for myself!" To them I say, "But who else deserves it more and who will appreciate it more?" Eating alone is not something to be ashamed of or avoided, like some secret shame. You want to get into the GLORY and luxury of eating in solitude. Many people would envy you the pleasure of your own uninterrupted company and the freedom to choose what *you* want to eat and when *you* want to eat it!

Affirmations About Eating Alone:

1. I, _____, am a worthwhile and pleasing person whether I am alone or with others.
2. When I am alone, I, _____, am with my best friend who loves and cares most for me.
3. I, _____, deserve the delicious meals that I fix and serve to myself.
4. When I, _____, eat alone, I am an honored and valued guest at the table.

5. I, _____, choose to eat in solitude to best appreciate the total flavor of my food.
6. I, _____, enjoy the time I take to prepare and eat the meals I have alone.
7. I, _____, am deeply nourished by the food I prepare and eat alone.
8. I, _____, can choose to sit at the table in silence or to meditate when I eat alone.
9. My meals eaten alone give me so much pleasure that I, _____, now eat much less and lose weight.
   My meals eaten alone give me so much pleasure that I, _____, now eat more and lose weight.
10. I, _____, look forward with pleasure to the luxury of a meal in solitude.

When You Go On a Binge

When and if you forget everything, find yourself going on a binge, eating when you don't want to eat, stuffing yourself and not experiencing any of it, hating yourself for it all— STOP! Acknowledge yourself for catching yourself before you ate *three* boxes of chocolates. Stop and think about God instead. Say "Oh, thank God I stopped myself now and I forgive myself!" Instead of thinking about how bad you were, forgive yourself.

Try thoughts like these:

I forgive myself for eating when I wasn't hungry.
I forgive myself for nibbling and not being conscious of what I was doing.
I forgive myself for being nervous.
I forgive myself for bringing myself down.
I forgive myself for going back to the ego.
I forgive myself for thinking it was wrong to eat this food.
I forgive myself for thinking I couldn't eat this food.
I forgive myself for not pleasing myself with this food.
I forgive myself for using this syndrome as a defense.

Then be willing to sit down calmly and handle what you were really covering up. Did you start to binge because of some fear? Did you binge because you wanted to prove some negative thought?

Remember the mind thinks and proves what it thinks. Whatever you think, your mind tries to prove is RIGHT. So whatever you believe to be true is whatever you created for yourself. Suppose you have the thought, "This diet will never work for me." To prove this thought, you will have to go back to the refrigerator and eat to prove that you can never get over this habit. You won't change until you change the negative thought into a positive one. You can start right now by thinking and creating for yourself this thought:

Everything works for me if I, _____, want it to.

Affirmations After a Binge:

1. I, _____, can choose the times when I will or will not eat.
2. When I am nervous or upset, I, _____, can handle the problem without eating.
3. My mind is creating only helpful, positive thoughts for me, _____.
4. I, _____, am pleasing to myself whether I binge out or avoid food.
5. I, _____, deserve to eat whatever food I want.
6. I, _____, can stop eating any food I want, even if it is only half eaten.
7. I, _____, eat only when my body needs food.
8. My body wants what is best for me, _____, and it will not betray me with foods that are harmful.
9. My body is helping me, _____, to solve my overweight problem.
10. This diet is working for me because I, _____, want it to.

Food Games

I finally confessed my nervousness about food to my friends Jim and Joan Morningstar in Milwaukee. They decided to help me out by laying out in front of me one of my favorite sinful foods—sausage. Joan cut six pieces for me, demonstrating that she was willing to sit there with me and watch me eat them and help me through my fear. I said I couldn't eat because I had too much fear. The only way I could eat the sausage was if we made up a real game about it. This game turned out to be hilarious.

First, we made up some instructions about what you could do with the sausage. Because I was so fearful of the supposed power of a sausage, we acted as if the sausage had a life and a will of its own. We made up some instructions as if the sausage was a thing and some as if it were alive. Next we wrote the instructions on paper and cut them into cards, with one instruction on each. Then we put the cards face down in a pile and took turns drawing one each. We had to follow the instruction on the card. Here are the instructions:

Eat two.
Throw one.
Love one.
Talk to one for five minutes.
Eat one.
Push one across the floor with your nose.
Feed one to someone else.
Have a fantasy with one.

Needless to say, after playing this game, I lost my fear of sausage. How can you be afraid of something you are laughing at? I laughed so much, I lost a couple of pounds right on the spot. And I got clear on sausage. The next day I ate lots of sausage and had no fear! So much for sausage and the Sausage Game.

You can make up your own game with any food that you fear. Perhaps your mind says the most "evil" foods are the ones with the most calories; therefore, you are afraid of them. If you have created these monstrous, fearsome foods, get ready to destroy their power with laughter!

Another day I made up a game called Changing the Meaning of Calories. Calories used to control me. I hated them and I feared them. I believed calories were delicious, invisible lumps of fat hiding in the foods I loved best. When I ate those foods, I took up the burden of those calories and they became visible on my body in rolls and bulges of flesh. Because this effect was something I created by my belief in my mind, I decided to uncreate it.

I decided I was going to see calories as units of energy my own body produces to burn up food and do other things. That is, calories aren't something out there waiting to get me. They are something my body in its own wisdom decides to make and use as it considers best. So I decided to think of calories as energy my body makes to keep me warm, make new skin and hair, run all the organs my body needs to stay healthy, and let me move freely to work, play, and love as I choose.

That afternoon I needed to sort through some mail, write a few letters, and do some laundry—none of which I felt very motivated to do. When I sat down to lunch, I decided to look at the food in this new way, seeing foods as units of energy I would gain power from. Now, food isn't calories to be feared, but fuel and energy. That's what I mean by fat is just stuck energy.

Affirmations About Food and Calories:

1. I, _____, can create my own ideas about what foods are safe or fattening for me.
2. I, _____, can laugh at any food without fear of getting fat.
3. No food is dangerous to me if I, _____, can laugh at it.
4. Foods want to be my friends if I, _____, will relax and let them.
5. I, _____, can choose to look at food and laugh without eating it.
6. I, _____, am a friend of calories because they do not make me fat.
7. I, _____, have never tasted, smelled, felt, or heard a calorie.
8. Calories cannot hurt me, _____, if I choose not to let them.
9. My body processes calories wisely for the many needs I, _____, have to live.
10. Calories give my body only power and energy, not fat.

The Forgiveness Diet

Perhaps your mind may still be addicted to thinking that it needs to diet from something or other. So why not make up a whole new kind of diet, one that doesn't have to do with giving up food or calories at all?

One day at the beach I was trying to help a friend who had a serious problem of overweight. She was very distraught and upset that day. At the time, I also wanted far more release on this subject for myself. I prayed about this for both of us and then picked up a book I had brought along that was a summary of *A Course in Miracles.*

I had been rebirthing this friend enough to know that part of her problem was that she was stuck in resentment. I found myself reading to her that Jesus had said: "Forgive seventy times seven." I wondered why he had said exactly that and what it really meant. I thought about it quite a while, seeking an answer.

I decided that maybe seventy times seven, which is 490, is how many forgiveness affirmations it would take to get serious about releasing the suppressed anger that one had had for some twenty or thirty years! Obviously, just saying one affirmation of forgiveness two or three times would never be enough to unlock the mind. Even seventy times would not be enough. Maybe seventy times seven would be enough.

Later my friend Jim from the Church of Religious Science Ministry in Seattle told me that seventy times seven means completion. I liked this idea and I liked the word. *Completion* doesn't mean ended or done with. It means filled up, with nothing lacking, or perfectly equipped and skilled. I knew then that I wanted completion. I wanted to help my friends and clients to have it. I wanted all of us to feel complete, free of guilt and fear.

I was willing to do anything to feel complete and keep from worrying. This time, I decided, I really mean it. So I sat there and made up a new diet. See if you don't agree it sounds a lot more fun than denying yourself food.

I thought that if you did something seventy times seven, it would show your intention was so high that you really meant it. You would be reprogramming your computer well enough for God to get that now you really, truly do mean it and you really, truly are ready. Then you would get all the energy you ever need to help you achieve that *permanent* result.

Obviously, when forgiveness is complete, there will be a flowing, fluid energy that is total love and it will be easy to guide your molecules to your exact desired weight. The molecules will simply respond to your mind immediately. But while you are stuck in hate and anger, your body will react like a naughty child and not obey your instructions.

So regularly every day, whenever I felt like it, I would sit down and write this affirmation: "I, Sondra, completely forgive my father." I wrote it seventy times each day for seven days. I did this affirmation at the typewriter because I can type very fast. But if I had not typed, I would have been totally willing to write it out by hand, which I sometimes did. I was thoroughly, totally willing to get off it.

When I first started this diet, I decided to run an experiment and eat anything I wanted. That idea scared me a little too much so I decided not to think about food at all. Only if I really felt hungry would I eat. I tried to separate food from dieting. Now I was dieting with words. I was feeding myself words and just playing around with food. This trick really worked for me!

After doing a set of seventy affirmations, I would get so high that I would just lie down and breathe in ecstacy. A few times I got a little scared because so much new energy was coming through me from God and love. I was not used to so much energy, but I relaxed in it and kept telling myself, "I am safe." Sometimes I would meditate on the affirmation, "It is now safe to completely forgive my father."

Then one night I ate baked potatoes with sour cream *and* fetucchine. I had no weight gain! Now I was free to eat when my body told me it needed food. I had totally forgiven my father, and my body and mind felt complete without eating.

Using the Forgiveness Diet

First Week:
This week, write one affirmation seventy times each day for seven days. You can do thirty-five in the morning and thirty-five in the evening. Use one that applies to you. I used this one, for example:

I, _____, *forgive my father completely.*

Second Week:
The following week write another affirmation seventy times each day for seven days. Here is the one that I used:

I, _____, *forgive my mother completely.*

Third Week:
The next week write this affirmation about yourself the same way, seventy times a day for seven days:

I, _____, forgive myself completely.

Fourth Week:
Now write this affirmation seventy times for seven days to release any trauma or anger about your own birth:

I, _____, forgive my obstetrician completely.

Constantly releasing energy in this way will produce miracles in your mind and body and life. All my friends and students who have tried it have also told me so.

Affirmations About Forgiveness:

1. I, _____, am ready to forgive myself now.
2. I, _____, am ready to forgive those I used to blame for wronging me for some reason.
3. It is safe for me, _____, to forgive myself now.
4. It is safe for me, _____, to forgive those I once blamed for wronging me.
5. I, _____, deserve and want completion now.
6. I, _____, am willing to do the affirmations as many times as I need to in order to gain completion.
7. Because I am feeding myself on words, I, _____, do not have to eat all the time.
8. I, _____, am ready to give up all my anger and resentment now.
9. I, _____, am ready to relax and accept the energy that is total love.
10. I, _____, can safely accept love for myself and offer forgiveness to myself and others.
11. I, _____, am now spiritually nourishing.
12. I, _____, allow the Holy Spirit to undo all my wrong thinking that keeps me stuck.

Affirmations for
The Only Diet There Is

A Contribution by Phil Laut

1. *I forgive myself for accepting food when I wanted love.*
2. *I am certain that there is enough food and love for me.*

For most people, one activity certain to produce parental approval was cleaning up your plate. Eating everything in front of you brought you praise and good feelings from adults. Eating can therefore be an emotional response you carry with you from childhood onward. As an adult, feelings of loneliness or rejection will frequently cause you to take an immediate trip to the refrigerator, a candy machine, or the nearest fast-food restaurant. Through eating, you hope to recapture that feeling of warmth and love that resulted from eating it all up when you were a child.

3. *I forgive my mother for her unwillingness to nourish me at birth and her attempts to overfeed me later.*

All of us have received conditioning about food. This conditioning was started at a very early age, at the age of a few minutes for some of us, and was repeated several times daily for many years. In many homes a mealtime is an emotion-charged event. The family gathers together to eat the food prepared by one family member as an expression of love. To reject the food is to reject the love of this food preparer. In many families, attendance at meals is mandatory. Admonitions to eat are usually accompanied by warnings of grave consequences if they are not carried out. Thus food and eating are emotion-packed topics.

4. *My body is safe whether I eat or not.*
5. *My body has a natural tendency toward health and beauty whether I eat or not.*

The people who preach the practice of eating three meals a day have never tried any other way of eating. There is no scientific evidence that eating three meals a day will enable anyone to stay healthy forever. I like the statement that doctors live on 75 percent of what we eat and their patients live on the other 25 percent.

6. *Because I am the one who knows the most about my body, it is easy for me to heal or change it.*

Food has nothing to do with weight. If overeating were the true cause of overweight, then everyone who overeats would be overweight. It is the thoughts and attitudes you have about yourself, about food, and about your body that cause overweight. Only by changing your thoughts and attitudes about yourself, about food, and about your body will you free yourself from the tyranny of endless worrying and endless dieting.

7. *I like my body, and the more I like it, the more lovable it becomes.*
8. *Because I created my body, it is easy for me to love it.*

An important first step in mastering your body is to love it, to love it exactly the way it is now. If you think disapproving thoughts about your body, you are telling your body that you do not think it is okay. Your body will act out those thoughts or commands by refusing to cooperate with you. If you cannot love your body the way it is, then this inability is an indication of the power your body has over you. Being able to love your body exactly as it is right now is the first step to mastering it.

9. *Everything I eat turns to health and beauty.*

The popularity of the belief that overeating causes overweight can, in some cases, make this become a self-fulfilling prophecy. If you have this belief, then I suggest that you start out with any good diet and combine it with the techniques in this book. This combination will enable you to seduce your mind away from the idea that food and weight have anything to do with each other and give you an opportunity to experience the truth. Even if you believe that food and weight are related, the relationship between the two has never been clearly formulated.

Let us assume, as an example, that you consume two pounds of food and liquids during an average day. Your intake adds up to 730 pounds a year, or slightly over SEVEN TONS in a twenty-year period. Medical science has never been clear as to whether your consumption would have to be reduced to FIVE TONS or to THREE TONS in order to lose the ten pounds you would like to shed.

Another scientific anomaly is that the fat-producing characteristics of food are measured in calories, which are units of heat. How calories produce fat has never been clear to me. It has always seemed that if a person ate extra calories above what he or she needed to live, the result should be that the person is warmer, rather than fatter!

10. *I have the right to say NO without losing people's love.*

Fear of sex is a common cause of overweight. For example, suppose you are a woman who thinks she is twenty pounds overweight and who receives three sexual propositions a month. You may be concerned that if you lose the weight you want to, then you will receive ten or twenty times as many sexual propositions. This is a frightening prospect if you are not certain of your right to say *no*.

11. *I no longer compare myself to others to know that I am good enough.*

Some women are never happy about the way their bodies look because they are constantly comparing them with the bodies of the models they see in *Vogue* or other fashion magazines. My version of the history of fashion photography may make this comparison a little easier for you to take.

At the time fashion photography started in the last century, it was fashionable for women to be buxom and hippy. When these women were used as fashion models, everyone spent more time ogling the models than they did looking at the clothes. Although this was very pleasant for the viewers, it did not sell clothes. Fashion designers then came up with the idea of using models who were so shapeless that they would force people to look at the garments they wore instead of the bodies in them. Perhaps this little tale will cause you to stop comparing yourself with fashion models.

12. *My body is an individual expression of me. I no longer have to work out family patterns in my body.*

For some people, it is simply part of the family tradition to be a little overweight. If your family has always told you that you looked just like your mother and if your mother was a little overweight, then your family was giving you instructions to look the same way. You can go on diets forever but they will not do you a bit of good until you change your belief that you are supposed to look like your mother.

Affirmations for The Only Diet There Is:

1. I, _____, forgive myself for accepting food when I wanted love.
2. I, _____, am certain that there is enough food and love for me.
3. I, _____, forgive my mother for her unwillingness to nourish me at birth and her attempts to overfeed me later.
4. My body is safe whether I, _____, eat or not.
5. My body has a natural tendency toward health and beauty whether I, _____, eat or not.
6. Because I, _____, am the one who knows the most about my body, it is easy for me to heal or change it.
7. I, _____, like my body and the more I like it, the more lovable it becomes.
8. Because I, _____, created my body, it is easy for me to love it.
9. Everything I, _____, eat turns to health and beauty.
10. I, _____, have the right to say *no* without losing people's love.
11. I, _____, no longer compare myself to others to know that I am good enough.
12. My body is an individual expression of me. I, _____, no longer have to work out family patterns in my body.

How the Birth Trauma is Related to Overweight

After having Rebirthed and counselled many people with overweight problems, I began to see the following thread: People who have had a rather violent, traumatic birth are more afraid in all the situations in their lives. They are afraid they will be "banged up," "hit," or practically killed because this is what they experienced when they were born. They were treated roughly, struck in order to make them breathe, and traumatized to the point where they feared they might die. The memory of these events, which is completely stored in their consciousness, is enough to keep them scared for the rest of their lives.

Often people who are so traumatized at birth have touching and love wired up with getting hurt. Later on in life, in order to protect themselves from being hurt again, from being beaten up, they put layers of fat around themselves. This protective flesh, they somehow believe, will keep them safe from danger. These extra layers of fat also act to keep these people from being loved, which seems to be a real danger to them too.

Many people have some strains of thinking that run this way. They may equate love and pain, love and death, or love and hurt together. These people may relax long enough to attract a partner, but then they are likely to resist that person's love or even try to get rid of the partner in order to feel safe. Although this fear may be suppressed at the beginning of the relationship, as time passes and the love gets more intense and brings up anything unlike itself, these fears from birth start surfacing. Unless the person is led into a situation like Rebirthing or some other method that processes the birth trauma, these fears from birth may come up so strongly that the only solution seems to be to leave a relationship that somehow brings them into consciousness. Love is like that— it brings up anything unlike itself.

This pattern of behavior became obvious to me when I tried out many varieties of the Truth Process about overweight on people while I was Rebirthing them. They would, with skillful questioning, get down to the real truth, which is "fear of being harmed." This fear was why they had to keep on the extra weight for protection, both as physical padding and as a means to keep potentially threatening love away.

I am very convinced, after five years of Rebirthing, that the birth trauma IS a factor in overweight. I have seen people frequently lose five pounds or more right before my eyes, just while breathing. Not only did they breathe out "heavy" thoughts, they also breathed out the fear that had caused them to put protective padding around themselves in the first place.

When people begin to study their birth, they are sometimes very surprised to find out that the events surrounding it were so rough and that the birth itself had such a profound, all-encompassing effect on their lives. They often go through a long period of resenting the way they were handled (or rather mishandled) at birth. They may want to blame the obstetrician or their mother for the pain they caused them at birth. Forgiveness affirmations and prayers are very helpful in coping with this resentment.

However the real healing of the birth trauma comes after you take TOTAL responsibility for creating everything in your life, including the kind of birth you created for yourself. Coming through with past life karma, for example, means you are responsible even for choosing your parents and for your conception, your time in utero, and your delivery. If you come through with full consciousness, as we now see that babies do, then you tend to set up your birth to be as you expect. Therefore your parents, the obstretrical team, and the others present at your birth respond to your energy as a being and to your thoughts. It does not matter that you are merely a newborn with a small body. You have very sophisticated thinking processes and you make very sophisticated decisions. These mental abilities are formed in the womb and even before. All our research has shown this to be true, as you can see by reading *Rebirthing in the New Age*.

However, the important idea here is not to focus on your past lives or even on whether they exist or not. The important thing is to get that you can't blame your overweight on others involved with your birth trauma because you have somehow set that up yourself. Understanding this, and being willing to learn more about it and accept it, does make it easier to clear up your weight problem. It is very hard to clear up any of your problems if you are stuck in blame.

Getting Rebirthed is the ultimate answer for me. Releasing one's birth trauma removes most of this fear and any remaining fear you will feel safe to handle by yourself. I always Rebirth myself during sex or massage. Letting yourself experience out your fear of death while having pleasure is a very high spiritual practice. That is why making love is communion with God and quite the opposite of anything sinful.

Affirmations About the Birth Trauma:

1. I, _____, forgive everyone at my birth for the way in which I was handled at birth.
2. I, _____, am ready to accept love free of thoughts of pain, hurt, or death.
3. With the help of God, I, _____, know I am safe in a world that wishes only good for me.
4. It is now safe for me, _____, to give up my extra weight.
5. I, _____, am now ready to feel safe in accepting love.
6. I, _____, am ready to accept responsibility for having chosen my parents and my family.
7. I, _____, am ready to accept the responsibility for having chosen the kind of birth I had.
8. I, _____, am ready to accept the responsibility for my overweight problem.
9. Because I, _____, have created my life and my overweight, I can also change them.
10. I, _____, am now ready to learn how to create the kind of life I truly want.

Breathing Exercises

At one time my mind was so conditioned that I believed I had to exercise to lose weight. Until I could integrate the thought that I could lose weight without exercising, I decided to do the easiest exercise I could think of. The easiest exercise I know of is to lie in bed and breathe deeply!

Whenever you feel full or uncomfortable after eating, just lie down and breathe a lot. Later on you can Rebirth yourself through any trying situation. Until then, you can simply lie down and breathe gently and deeply. Inhale God and love; exhale fear and discomfort. Deep breathing will help you to transmute the food quickly into energy instead of fat. If your tummy is upset, breathing will make you feel better because chances are that queasy feeling is due to the guilty, negative thoughts you had while eating, rather than the food itself. If you were suppressing anger during the meal, that can also cause your stomach to feel uncomfortable or too full. Breathing deeply will help you with suppressed anger because you can release it on each exhale. For the best available instructions on breathing, see *Rebirthing in the New Age*.

Whenever you breathe deeply, you are taking in more aliveness and therefore more thinness. I have had many people lose five pounds or more during a Rebirth. One woman set a record during one of my Loving Relationships Training classes in New York. During the two and a half day training she stood up, yelled all her feelings out, and breathed and cried a lot. In one sharing she dumped thirty-three pounds of negative mental mass!

Another easy exercise to lose weight is to go outside in your car or into the woods and yell. Yelling out your anger into space usually will lead you spontaneously into a period of deep, rich breathing. It is hanging onto your anger that makes you heavy.

The key exercise that I encourage during this diet, and at all other times of stress, is deep breathing. It makes an amazing difference in your life when you come to understand that you don't have to stuff food into yourself when you are nervous, angry, or sad. Instead of eating, you can lie down and breathe deeply, letting go of these heavy emotions. To be quite honest and to speak from the bottom of my heart, I know there isn't ANY problem that cannot be cleared up through changing thoughts, forgiveness, love, breathing, Rebirthing, and prayer. Deep breathing is like a deep cleansing that purifies your body of negative, threatening feelings as it nourishes you with God and love.

Affirmations About Breathing Exercises:

1. I, _____, am ready to accept that I do not need to do physical exercises in order to lose weight.
2. With each breath I draw, I, _____, inhale God and love to nourish me.
3. With each breath I let out, I, _____, exhale fear, doubt, and discomfort.
4. I, _____, can control my feelings of stomach upset through deep breathing and awareness.

5. I, _____, can deal with my known and suppressed anger by breathing it out.
6. My body obeys the commands that I, _____, give it now.
7. I, _____, deserve to be free of anger and nourished by love.
8. When I am emotionally upset, I, _____, can solve my problem without eating.
9. My body relaxes and my emotions calm down when I, _____, breathe deeply and tell them to.
10. With the help of God, I, _____, can handle any problem through deep breathing and prayer.

How the Parental Disapproval Syndrome Affects Your Thinking About Food

One of your earliest attempts to please your parents may well be linked with that familiar domestic battleground—the dinner table. Think about your early, and probably unsuccessful, efforts to feed yourself, sit up straight at the table, and above all, eat everything that someone else had put on your plate! Mealtimes were also the occasions when you got to tell in front of everyone what you had done wrong that day. So food is associated with negativity and disapproval. Whenever you eat, alot of "circuits are triggered" around disapproval. You can also keep the parental disapproval syndrome going (which is a habit) by eating when and what you think you shouldn't and then disapproving of yourself as if you were your own angry parent.

Affirmations About the Parental Disapproval Syndrome:

1. My parents love me no matter what I, _____, eat.
2. My parents love me for what I, _____, eat and what I don't eat.
3. I, _____, feel good about what I eat.
4. I, _____, no longer fear disapproval about what I eat.
5. Sitting at the dinner table is a source of love, fellowship, and harmony.

Heal Death and Lose Weight

We have learned in Rebirthing that overweight is really just stuck energy due to fear. The fear comes from a belief that something bad could happen to you, that there is something outside of you, more powerful than you are, that you must watch out for. This fear comes from a lack of understanding of the truth and from doubting God. The ultimate fear is that something terrible could happen and you could die. Death is the stronghold of all fears.

Suppose someone traced down each fear you have by asking you, "And what would happen then? And what would happen after that?" The last fear to come out would be, "I might die." This is how overweight is really connected to the belief in death. Now you can see why the only diet that will work permanently, freeing you from worrying or watching what you eat, is the diet that handles that fear.

The awareness of physical immortality gives one the certainty of being in control of his or her own body. The fear is worked out gradually as you learn that you are always safe in the universe if you choose not to die. *A Course in Miracles* says: Death is the result of the thought we call the Ego; Death is the result of this predominant thought: "Death is inevitable." Thoughts create results; believing that thought causes death. As you become more and more certain of this fact, you can drop any extra weight you are carrying, which is just a fake protection anyway. Now you understand why the following technique will be a powerful way to lose weight without dieting.

Sit across from a friend who understands affirmations, or better yet, one who understand Rebirthing. Otherwise pick someone you feel very safe with. Look that person in the eyes and say, "I am safe and immortal right now." Then notice the incredible feelings and sensations going on in your body as you say this statement and breathe deeply. I have lost weight just sitting and using this technique!

The other step in losing weight is totally loving your body. Love your body as much as God loves the earth—eternally. Now you may find this hard to do if you feel your body isn't the way it is supposed to be. You may protest, "How can I love my body when it isn't doing what I want it to do? How can I love my body when it isn't the way I want it to be?" In fact, you may be very angry with your body and yourself over your appearance. You may think it is impossible ever for you to love your body.

There is one missing link in your thinking here, however. Your body IS doing what you want it to. It is being what you want it to be. You did want to be the size and shape you are for some deeper reason. Therefore, love your body for serving you. There is a great lesson here for you to learn from your overweight.

I got through this transition by realizing that during my period of overweight, I was feeling fear and my extra pounds protected and padded me so that I would feel safe. I realized that until I worked out my fear, I was a lot better off taking it out on my body with a few extra pounds than with the frequent auto accidents I was having at that time.

One Thanksgiving Day, I was Rebirthing myself in the bathtub. I made a decision to turn my body over to God and to trust that it would come out beautiful. I could never surrender my body to God before because I was afraid God would take it away and I would die. I believed God caused all death. (As Leonard Orr says, "Man has always hated God for putting him in a closed universe from which there was no escape of death.") By that time I knew definitely that I was in charge of my own life and death and, if I trusted myself, it was safe to surrender my body to myself and God. That was the turning point in my mastery of my body.

The last important part of loving your body is to pleasure it. Pleasure it more than you have ever imagined doing before. Give it lots of massage, sex, and tender loving care. All this pleasure might arouse a lot of fear at first because as a result of their birth trauma most people have the belief that pain follows pleasure. When they let themselves have a lot of pleasure, the fear that something terrible will happen is always imminent on a deep level. This fear keeps them from surrendering. The way out of this box is to breathe out the fear while having pleasure. The thought one can have here is *pleasure* leads *to more pleasure* and *pleasure increases my safety and aliveness.*

The final thought is: Let your overweight teach you everything! Let it teach you what your fears are. Let it teach you the mastery of your body and of physical immortality. Let it teach you how to become a Spiritual Master! You are one, as Jesus has said. Isn't it time for you to become fully aware?

Affirmations About Healing Death:

1. I, _____, am safe in the universe because I am protected by God's endless love.
2. I, _____, am safe in the universe because I choose not to die.
3. Death cannot conquer me, _____, because I am immortal now if I choose to be.
4. I, _____, can lose my extra weight if I choose because I do not need it to protect me from death.
5. I, _____, love and admire my body as it is.
6. My body deserves all the pleasures I, _____, can provide for it.
7. My body is pleasing to me, _____, and attractive to others.
8. I, _____, am in charge of my own life and death.
9. I, _____, trust myself and God to love and care for my body.
10. I, _____, turn my body and all my other problems over to God.
11. I, _____, am safe and immortal right now.
12. The safer and more alive I, _____, feel the less extra weight I'll have.

Part Three

Facing the Truth

Are you truly ready to give up this problem?
Are you ready to give up this problem now?

If your answer is *no,* you have to face the situation you are in. This book will not work for you at this time. Put it down and read it again later when you are ready.

If you are ready, then you must face the truth about yourself. Doing so can be uncomfortable. At times you may cry or get angry about it. You may not like hearing the truth. Few people do. I understand that because I have been there myself.

The following pages give some examples of what has kept other people from getting off it. These are typical causes of what kept them from losing weight. What others have learned about themselves can help you learn more about yourself. If you don't want to face the truth about yourself, then you might as well not read the next few pages. You might as well go back to your stuckness.

I suggest you read the following pages and face yourself once again with the truth. This process is called a Final Clearing. By working through it, you will have a last and final chance to look at the reasons for your problem, the payoffs that make you want to hold on to it, and the deeper fears behind your problem.

Final Clearing

Here is some first aid for a problem of overweight or for any other problem. This aid is a three-part process. In each part you will first see what other people have said about their problems, some of which may also apply to you. Then you must face yourself and list the reasons for your behavior.

To begin part one, read the explanations below that people have given for holding on to their problem, whatever it was. As you read, stop after each reason and ask yourself if it could also apply to you.

These are my reasons for holding onto this problem:

EXAMPLES:

1. I don't love God enough. I love my problems more.
2. I don't believe that I can change my weight by my mind.
3. I think it is impossible to lose weight without dieting.
4. I don't want to get over my problem because I love to complain.
5. This problem gets me a lot of sympathy and attention from others.
6. I can use this problem to be angry at myself.

7. It is a sin for me to love my body; therefore, I must hate it.
8. It would be too good to be true if I could lose weight with a thought alone.
9. This process invalidates all my former belief systems.
10. If this process worked, what my mother said would be wrong and I can't make her wrong.
11. Who am I to think I am so powerful?
12. I don't know how to handle this feeling of helplessness.
13. If I were too beautiful, somebody would want sex with me.
14. If I were my exact desired weight I would have everything, and that much would be dangerous.
15. If I were my exact desired weight I would be perfect and that must be wrong.
16. I hang on to this problem because I don't want to get better.
17. I don't want to get better because then I would be perfect and people would be jealous.
18. I don't want to be my exact desired weight because then I would have everything.
19. I don't want to have everything because I would not know what to do without a problem.
20. I don't want to be perfect because this way I can hate God and prove life does not work.

Now face your own reasons for holding on to your problem. Start your own truth list below. You may use any of the reasons above that are yours as well. But add to them the reasons that you alone know apply to you.

These are my reasons for holding on to this problem:

1. _____
2. _____
3. _____
4. _____
5. _____
6. _____
7. _____
8. _____
9. _____
10. _____

Any problem can also seem to have some payoffs, in other words: what do I get out of keeping it. Here are some of the payoffs that other people have admitted they got for not giving up their problem. As you read them, pause after each one to ask yourself if it could apply to you as well.

These are my payoffs for having this problem:

EXAMPLES:

1. I get to complain.
2. I get to have problems to work on.
3. I get to think I am not good enough.
4. I get to have an excuse for any failure.
5. I get to keep men/women away.
6. I get to create a conflict to avoid joy.
7. I get to be right about my belief system.
8. I get to make my mother wrong because she said you had to be thin.
9. I get to avoid sex because no one would want this body.
10. I get to occupy my time by worrying.
11. I get to show that I am not perfect.
12. I get to have others worry about me.

13. I get to have doubts about everything.
14. I get to prove nobody wants me.
15. I get to have a reason to give up and die.
16. I get an excuse to hate God.
17. I get to lie about myself.
18. I get to avoid what I could be.
19. I get to receive help and attention from people.
20. I get to be angry at myself.

What are my fears about giving up this problem:

EXAMPLES:

1. I'm afraid that without it I wouldn't have anything to talk about.
2. I'm afraid that without it I would be beautiful and this must be dangerous.
3. I'm afraid of how much power I would have if I gave this up and got thin with my mind.
4. I'm afraid of giving up this problem because then I would have everything.
5. I'm afraid of having everything because then nobody would like me.
6. I'm afraid of giving up this problem because I would be clear without it.
7. I'm afraid of being clear because I would be like God.
8. I'm afraid of being like God because I would be punished. I am supposed to be a sinner and unlike God.
9. I'm afraid of giving up this problem because I would die without it.
10. I'm afraid I would die if I did not have problems.
11. I'm afraid of not having this problem because I would be complete without it and completion equals death.
12. I'm afraid that I will die if I eat. I also fear I will die if I don't eat.

13. I'm afraid of feeling too wonderful if I don't have a problem.

14. I'm afraid that people could not relate to me if I felt wonderful because I did not have this problem. People love misery and so they would leave me alone.

15. I'm afraid of giving up my problem because I love the pain it brings.

Now make up a list of the fears you have about giving up your problem. You can begin by using any from the list above that also apply to you.

These are my fears about giving up this problem:

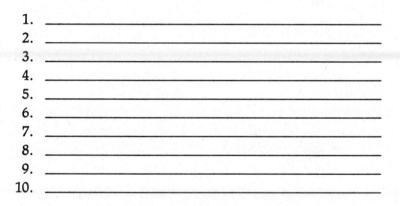

1. _____
2. _____
3. _____
4. _____
5. _____
6. _____
7. _____
8. _____
9. _____
10. _____

Fasting

Every now and then it is valuable to experiment with fasting to produce a greater mastery over your mind and body. The body does not need to be fed on a regular schedule three or more times a day at certain times unless you buy into that belief. If the body uses food for pleasure and energy, then it should be allowed to determine when it should have food based on its own needs. Think how many times you have been involved in some pleasurable activity or project and "forgotten" to eat. You didn't forget to eat; you didn't need to eat. Your body in its own wisdom was so involved that it was not interrupted by some other routine, such as a mealtime. Listen to the wisdom of your body.

As children, we chose to eat naturally when our bodies needed food. But adults conditioned us to eat when it was convenient for them to prepare and serve us food. As adults, we can again choose our own times to eat or not to eat at all. The last reason for eating should be because you looked at the clock and your mind told your body this is a time to eat. I have actually met Breatharians who know that food is a belief system that was made up. They do not buy into that belief system and they live on the elements and light of God.

Fasting will teach you a lot about your food neuroses. Through unconscious habit or conditioned avoidance, we tend to eat some foods frequently and almost totally ignore others. If left alone, our food choices could become very limited. Abstaining from all foods, those you like as well as those you ignore or dislike, can wipe the slate clean. Then you can start over to select foods with a greater freedom from past experiences and neuroses.

Fasting will give you new appreciations about the texture, color, smell, taste, and sound of food. For many people, eating is an activity to be gotten through. For them it is just a matter of fill the plate, feed the face, stuff the stomach. Meanwhile they are talking or arguing, reading, or watching television. All these activities are occupying more of their consciousness than the food they are eating. But fasting from food allows you to feast on your memories of food. How would you describe the essence of a ripe orange to someone who had never eaten one? How does it look? How does it feel and smell as you peel it? How does it sound and taste as you eat it? These sensations become fresh and new when you experience them again, like a child, for the first time.

A number of fasts are available, some of which begin with a total elimination of all food and liquids and some with a gradual elimination of certain foods each day. I recommend the Master Cleaser Fast juice fasts. A good book on the subject is *Are You Confused* by Paavo Airola.

More Food for Thought

Instead of praying for the end of your problem, pray for the release of your fear of giving it up! After all, you are hanging on to your overweight problem because of the fear of giving it up. Without this fear, you would have given it up and moved on long ago. So don't look only at your problem, seeking somehow to end it as your goal. Look around and behind your problem to the fear that locks it into your ego and your life.

Seeing the truth about anything heals it. Worry and fear about something can fill you with negative feelings that keep you from enjoying life, even from planning and acting in your own best interests. So face these unknowns in yourself, your worst fears and worries. Then set them aside, forgiving yourself for the grief you have caused yourself.

When you love God more than your problem, you will be healed. Your problem may be an excuse for you to focus on yourself and to get others to do the same. It is an endless chorus of me, me, me. By thinking about your problem and yourself so much, you have little time to meditate or think about God. You may not realize it, but you are using your problem to shut out God. To be healed, you must give up your self-hate, a kind of twisted self-love, and surrender to the love of God. As St. Francis of Assisi said: In order to find yourself, you must first lose yourself.

Whenever you start thinking about fat or your problem, STOP. Think about God instead. That is, give up your negative thoughts about yourself and your problem. Shut off the ego. Meditate, use affirmations, and turn your thoughts to God, the source of all help and healing.

Food and Spirituality

I have seen people try everything in order to lose weight. I have seen them try everything, that is, but prayer. Through prayer it is possible to achieve the weight that is in perfect harmony with God's pattern for your body. Other programs of dieting have a major flaw. They are only a temporary remedy. There is always that terrible chance the weight will be regained because the CAUSE was not healed.

I suggest you start this program by asking for divine guidance. Reverence for God is spiritual nourishment. Once you have spiritual nourishment, you will feel continuously satisfied. You will naturally eat less and you can even reach the point at which you eat as the spiritual masters do. They eat only for the sheer pleasure of eating when they feel like it.

If you love and respect your body spiritually, you will avoid overeating and overdrinking naturally. But until you have completely mastered your body to the point at which you can transmute all food into light, I advise you to be temperate. If you are really wise, you will take only the food and drink that you know is suitable for you.

The body's desire for food has its roots in the soul's need for spiritual substance. Affirm that your appetite and assimilation of food are in divine order. Perhaps your overweight is due to an imbalance between your inflow and outflow of energy. Somewhere the fat person is blocking on giving and receiving so that these two flows are not correctly balanced.

Because your body is intelligently equipped to choose, digest, and assimilate the right food for its own maintenance, it helps to pray for God to instruct you in these matters. Expect guidance. Expect the perfect pattern for your own body to come to its complete expression. Every gland, organ, and cell will respond to your thoughts that are in truth. God will actually help you select your food and lead you to the right people to help you release negativity and to get healed.

Your body is nourished by thought substances as well as by food and the light of God. Because your thoughts determine your desires, your appetite will lead you to foods that correspond with your thoughts. If food suggests fatness to you, however, then what you eat will largely be converted into fat. People who are slender or even underweight have the thought, "No matter how much I eat, I can't gain weight." Their bodies follow their thought pattern and they stay very thin.

Many overweight people seek to control their bodies through various food diets and exercise plans. But *control* is not the answer; letting go into God is the answer. You must be ready to trust God enough to turn over the control of your body with confidence that a plan of perfection exists for you. If you want to transform your body, you must gain freedom from these and all the other limited thoughts of the past. Everything that is out of order in your body is due to some false, negative thought that you have.

Ask for a release of all your negative thoughts and your destructive habits. Never indulge in worry, hate, fear, or pain while you are eating. Every time I have done this I have gained weight, regardless of how few calories were supposedly in the food I ate. Affirming the presence of God while you eat and dedicating the food to the service of God changes everything. Bless every mouthful and experience the food as you eat, rather than talking, complaining, and worrying at meals.

Praying over food is always a good idea. Food that is spiritually blessed takes on the substance of the Spirit. You can simply say, "I bless this food to the building of my body and I bless the pleasure I receive from it in the name of _____." (Name any spiritual leader you wish.)

The best and most permanent diet I know is a spiritual diet. Faith is the most important nourishment of all. Instead of counting calories, which keeps you stuck in old habits of thinking, spend the time studying spiritual truth. I suggest you make up your own spiritual diet of daily prayers. This can be a lot of fun and is very rewarding. Check into God's reducing clinic, which is much easier and cheaper than the commercial alternatives!

Here is a spiritual diet I suggest you try for a week, or you can prepare one of your own. The diet consists of an affirmation and a prayer of thanksgiving for each day.

Using the Spiritual Diet:

Day 1:
I, _____, ask for spiritual guidance to direct my way of eating.
For the divine help and spiritual guidance I have received, I give thanks.

Day 2:
I, _____, turn my body over to a higher power and ask for a divine blessing upon it.
For the spiritual care and protection I have been given, I give thanks.

Day 3:
I, _____, now choose only the foods and liquids that are suitable for my body.
For the spiritual direction I have been given in selecting correct foods, I give thanks.

Day 4:
I, _____, desire freedom from worry, tension, and fear while I am eating.
For the pleasure and relaxation I enjoy about food and eating, I give thanks.

Day 5:
I, _____, know that my appetite for food and my assimilation are in tune with the divine order.
For the improved balance I now experience in my intake and outake of energy, I give thanks.

Day 6:

I, _____, can now eat less food because I am nourished by the light of God.

For the spiritual nourishment I now receive that sustains me, I give thanks.

Day 7:

I, _____, now expect the perfect pattern for my body to come into its complete expression according to the divine plan.

For the freedom from my past negative thoughts and the transformation of my body, I give thanks.

The Atonement

Because you bought this book, you must have had courage. Since you've read this far, you must have had the courage to GET OFF IT! You must have had the courage to think about giving up your food case. You should acknowledge yourself for your bravery. Stop beating yourself up with your neuroses about food and start acknowledging yourself for thinking about giving it up.

Perhaps overweight is not your problem and you bought this book for another reason. You may have known intuitively that the method in this book applies to other problems as well as food. Perhaps on some level you knew that the Forgiveness Diet was in this book and that it would work for you. Then I acknowledge you for the courage you had to buy this book, face your problem, and want to do something about it.

To all of you I say, reading this book is one thing; applying it is another. You can read it and just forget it, or you can read it and actually use it. You, and only you, make the important next decision. Will you do the Forgiveness Diet?

You might say "no" and walk away.

You might say, "Yes, it sounds like a good idea," but then never do it.

You might say, "it sounds like such a good idea that I am going to do it," and then you still might not do it.

Or you might say, "It sounds as if it will work. I am going to do it." And then you actually DO it.

In which category are you? It depends on how much you desire healing. If you really mean that you want to be healed of your condition, then you will probably try anything that has worke⁻ for others. You will eventually try until you succeed in finding what works for you. When you are finally ready to get off your problem completely, you will find the thing to heal you and it will work. When you are completely ready to be healed, healing will happen one way or another. You could, however, have too much fear to be healed completely or miraculously. Because you think that your defense mechanisms protect you, you hang on to them. But defense mechanisms, like overweight or smoking, actually produce only more fear. As a result, you think you need more defense and you get more stuck.

The only thing that has ever worked for the tough, stuck condition that I had, was *God.* When I finally got healed of my food case after trying many things, I realized that what had done it was a lot of prayer and thinking about God. I was willing to do anything to be completely healed, even to "risk" trusting God completely. Because my ego thought somehow that was some kind of risk, I took longer than necessary to get myself healed. I turned to *A Course In Miracles* once again in frustration and it began to work. I had surrendered, or surrendered as much as I could at the time. Shortly after Thanksgiving 1980, I came up with this affirmation, or I should say, I finally allowed this affirmation to come through me.

"I allow the Holy Spirit to undo all of my wrong thinking."

This is the Atonement. The Atonement is the correction. The correction of your limiting crummy thoughts and the correction of the ego. This correction is what you must want. Your food case, or whatever case you have, is a result of your crummy thoughts. It is a result of the ego, which is like the devil. In a way when you are saying *no, no, no* to your own case, to your own negative thoughts, to your own bad habits, to your own stuckness and lack of progress, you are saying *no* to your ego. Therefore you are saying *yes* to God. You are saying, I am willing to be filled with God rather than with this. Then you will be healed.

The ego will not give you the tools to heal yourself because its extinction would be near. The ego will try to rear its ugly head and tell you that you should go back to worrying about food or whatever problem you have that keeps you out of peace. You will be tempted many times by the devil, which is your case or your ego, to indulge in negative thinking and in hopelessness.

How is your faith? Can you go for peace? Do you believe you can have peace of mind about food or your problem? If you say *no* to this question, how can you heal yourself? You must start with faith.

Overweight and underweight are similar to any other disease. You must get over your fear of not having the condition before you can expect a miracle, a healing, of the condition. The Spirit will not add to your fear. Thus the Spirit cannot heal you until you work out your fear of healing. This is important. If you do not understand what I mean, do not worry about it. What matters is that you forgive yourself for creating this mess and that you get over your fear of not having the condition that brings you down.

Therefore I recommend you to trust God and to offer your case or condition to the Holy Spirit and make the following affirmations:

It is completely safe for me, _____, to give up this condition (overweight, pain, or any suffering). It is completely safe to let God in completely. It is safe because God is love and God is life.

Because I was the thinker who thought that God was something to be feared and that God caused death, I, _____, am also the thinker who can now think that God is peace, love, and safety and that God increases life.

Because I, _____, no longer fear God, and I know God does not kill people, it is safe for me to pray to God about my problem and to expect God to help me with it.

I, _____, allow the Holy Spirit to undo all my wrong thinking.

Weight Affirmations

Again and again this book has stressed the importance of changing your thinking before you can expect to change your body. Your weight does not depend on whether you eat more or less food. What you eat does not harm you; what you believe about food is what harms you. Food does to your body only what you instruct it to do, thus seducing your subconscious. Here are some general affirmations about weight to help you further reshape your thought processes, and through them, your body.

1. My body automatically processes whatever food I, _____, take in to maintain my perfect weight and health.
2. My body is perfect when I, _____, weigh _____ pounds and wear a size _____.
3. My desired weight is _____ pounds, whether I, _____, eat or not.
4. I, _____, like my body and the more I like it, the more lovable it becomes.

5. Since I, _____, love my body, it now cooperates with my mind to maintain my desired weight.

6. My body has the capacity to transmute food automatically into light and love.

7. Everything I, _____, eat turns to health and beauty and my weight remains the same.

8. Everything I, _____, eat turns into my healthy and well-proportioned body at my desired weight.

9. Calories are not in charge of me. I, _____, am in charge of my weight and my body.

10. I, _____, have the right to lose weight whether it pleases my parents or not.

11. As long as I, _____, am maintaining my perfect weight, I am eating enough.

12. I, _____, will be healthy regardless of what I eat and weigh.

13. Everything I, _____, eat is good for me or I would not put it into my body.

14. I, _____, have the right to enjoy what I am eating in full view of everyone.

15. There is no longer any connection between what I, _____, eat and what I weigh.

16. I, _____, now feel good about myself whether I eat or not.

17. I, _____, never worry about gaining weight any more.

18. I, _____, no longer fear being overweight.

19. It is safe for me, _____, to be my ideal weight.

20. I, _____, deserve to be my ideal weight now.

Forgiveness Affirmations

If you are stuck in resentment, your mind is locked into old patterns of hate and worry. This bitterness against yourself and others retains the burden of hate and anger in your body. You must free your mind of this resentment if you are to free your body of its weight. Only then can you experience the slimness and freed energy that comes from total love. These affirmations will offer you some additional help in gaining that freedom to be thin.

1. I, _____, forgive my mother completely for what she taught me about food.
2. I, _____, forgive my parents for the tension they gave me about meals and eating.
3. I, _____, forgive those who were unkind to me about my weight problem.
4. I, _____, no longer resent _____. I forgive him/her completely.
5. I, _____, am ready to give up blaming others for my problem.

6. I, _____, now forgive myself completely.

7. I, _____, forgive myself for taking so long to stop hating myself.

8. I, _____, will continue to forgive _____ daily until I achieve my exact, desired weight.

9. I, _____, no longer blame food for my weight problem. I take the responsibility to forgive.

10. I, _____, give thanks that my food illusions and my weight illusions are disappearing.

11. It is safe for me, _____, to give up this weight syndrome in my mind.

12. I, _____, do not need to punish myself with this problem anymore.

13. I, _____, am now willing to experience the joy of being without this problem.

14. I, _____, have total peace of mind on this subject now.

15. It is now safe and pleasurable for me, _____, to be in my body totally.

16. I, _____, no longer use food or my body to beat myself up because I now use food and my body for pleasure.

17. I, _____, am willing to give up resentment and worrying completely.

18. I, _____, can handle all the energy that will be freed up by letting go of my food and body hangups.

19. Every time I, _____, slide backward and get nervous, I stop and think about God instead.

20. I, _____, nourish myself so much with God I don't think about food.

Eating Affirmations

Eating can and should be seen as just one of many pleasurable and sensual experiences available to you. It can be enjoyed alone or with others, in private or in public, and at almost any time you choose! By now, I hope you have set aside any tension or resentment about eating you may have had left over from childhood mealtimes. Through eating alone you have learned to experience the full enjoyment of eating, of all the textures, colors, sounds, smells, and especially the many tastes of foods. You know that food is available for your nourishment and pleasure. Food is not fattening for you if you so instruct your body.

To help you enjoy eating, I recommend the following affirmations. Now, enjoy your freedom to eat and enjoy eating!

1. I, _____, can eat and be happy without worry.
2. I, _____, can eat or not eat as I choose.
3. I, _____, eat small amounts of foods that are very pleasurable to me.
4. I, _____, eat only for pure celebration, pleasure, and ceremony.
5. My eating contributes to my aliveness, joy, and health.

6. I, _____, love myself in the presence of food.

7. I, _____, can eat any amount I want without any undesirable results.

8. Food does not hurt me unless I, _____, think it does.

9. I, _____, am highly pleasing to my grandparents and my parents whatever I eat.

10. Food is for the pleasure of eating and I, _____, deserve to enjoy it.

11. I, _____, do not have to eat just because everyone else is eating.

12. When I do eat, I, _____, eat only when I am relaxed.

13. I, _____, like to eat sitting down and undistracted by other people or activities.

14. I, _____, pay attention to the experience when I am eating.

15. I, _____, eat only what I want to eat.

16. I, _____, don't judge whether I should eat by time or habit; I eat only for fun.

17. I, _____, consciously choose what to eat and when to eat it.

18. I, _____, am able to eat whatever I want whenever I want to.

19. After I eat, I, _____, am happy, releaxed, and freed in my energy.

20. Everything I, _____, eat is nourishing to my body and soul and never harms me.

Final Affirmations

The affirmations below touch on all the topics and problems you have worked through during this process—weight, food, eating, fasting, love, sex, birth, death, forgiveness, and spirituality. At some time you may find yourself discouraged about your weight or other problems or your lack of progress toward a goal you have chosen. You may be tempted to fill up on food or worry or depression. Instead of taking on any of these burdens, use some of these affirmations. These are the last I can offer you.

1. I, _____, have the power to be the weight I desire.
2. I, _____, have the right to feel good about myself regardless of how I look or what I weigh.
3. My abdomen feels relaxed, calm, and thin at all times.
4. I, _____, feel very good in my body, especially in the midsection.
5. My body is now free of any tension and I, _____, feel good everywhere.
6. My body no longer causes me, _____, any concern.

7. I, _____, weigh _____ pounds no matter what I eat.

8. My metabolism is responding to the new instructions that I, _____, am giving it.

9. I, _____, am now relaxed and happy around food.

10. I, _____, love food and I know that it cannot harm me.

11. I, _____, am never bothered by food any more.

12. My thoughts about food, if I have any, are of its goodness.

13. Everything I, _____, eat is nourishing to my body and soul and never harms me.

14. Eating makes me feel safe. I, _____, also feel safe if I don't eat.

15. The foods that I, _____, eat are very pleasurable to me and I enjoy eating.

16. That which is pleasurable to me, _____, no longer has any undesirable consequences.

17. The more I, _____, experience pleasure from eating, the more attractive I become.

18. I, _____, approve of myself for eating. If I don't approve of eating, I don't do it.

19. I, _____, am a thin man/woman who can sit and eat slowly and stop before I am full.

20. I, _____, feel good whether I eat or not.

21. It doesn't matter to others or to me if I, _____, eat or not.

22. I, am gradually and spontaneously giving up food without worry or effort.

23. I, _____, am fully aware of what I eat and when I eat so that I no longer eat out of habit or to stuff my feelings.

24. I, _____, can fast as long as I want without any undesirable results.
25. I, _____, have given up the desire to eat.
26. I, _____, deserve all the attention and love I can get without having to perform for it.
27. I, _____, enjoy being attractive.
28. I, _____, am a masculine, sexy man.
    I, _____, am a feminine, sexy woman.
29. God created my body for me, _____, to use to win a kind and loving partner.
30. I have the right to use my body to win the kind of partner I, _____, want.
31. I, _____, have given up all resentment and fear associated with my experiences at birth.
32. I, _____, no longer blame my mother or the hospital staff for the trauma I experienced at birth.
33. I, _____, am ready to accept responsibility for having created the birth I experienced.
34. I, _____, am ready to accept the joys of love without fear of pain or death.
35. I, _____, no longer need to protect myself from death with extra bodyweight.
36. I, _____, stay young and become more attractive with more and more wonderful energy.
37. I, _____, am willing to stop blaming myself and others for my problems.
38. I, _____, deserve to be safe and happy, free of worry about my problem.
39. It is safe for me, _____, to give up hate and fear and to accept feeling good.
40. Because I think about God, I, _____, no longer think about food or my problem.
41. There is no problem that I, _____, with God's help, cannot resolve through deep breathing and prayer.

Part Four

What Is Eating?

Elsewhere in this book you have met some of the people who have helped me as I worked out my own healing and my plan for this book. They have shared their understandings and ideas with me, questioning and inspiring me. Sometimes what these teachers have *not* said or explained has affected me as much as what they have said. Now I would like to share some of my experiences of learning from them with you.

One of my teachers has been Robert Rosellini, a master chef. Thanks to him and his profound knowledge of his subject, I was finally able to complete this book, which had been blocked for about a year. At 3:00 a.m. a "Zen" talk with him finally released my mind, and I was healed. As you can understand, he is a special and significant person in my life.

Allow yourself now to transcend the past completely and prepare to have your experience of food and the body transformed. Let me take you into Robert's space, which I am sure you will find more than refreshing. Because my good friend and co-trainer Fred Lehrman had introduced Robert to me, I have asked him to introduce Robert to you.

Beyond Nourishment: Food as Meditation

by Fred Lehrman

In 1973, Grand Master Cheng Man-ch'ing, venerable Chinese teacher of the Five Excellences of Painting, Calligraphy, Medicine, Classic Texts, and the Martial Arts, told me of a Taoist Master under whom he had studied as a young man. This monk had developed some unusual powers. He wore the same thin cotton robe in every season, his body remaining cool in summer and warm in winter. He never bathed, yet his skin and hair were always shining, clean, and smelled sweetly. He drank only water, ate not at all, and was never seen asleep. He was regarded as Immortal by those who came to know him.

Once a year, on a special holiday, this monk would meet with a group of his peers for a day-long feast. From morning till sunset, these men would sit and devour course after course of rich food and wine. Their appetite and capacity seemed endless. The young Cheng Man-ch'ing observed this with perplexity.

On the following day, he approached his teacher with a question: "Master," he said, "how is it possible for you to consume so much after fasting for so long?"

The monk replied: "I do not eat that food. If I ate that food, I would die."

I tell this story as a way of introducing my friend Robert Rosellini to these pages. Robert is a master in the art of creating transformation through the dining experience. He has studied the best restaurants of Europe and has abstracted the subtle balance of timing, attitude, tone and decor within which to set the repast at the perfection of its visual and culinary potential. At his restaurant, Rosellini's Other Place in Seattle, Washington, his staff produces dinners in a relaxed and perfectly coordinated ballet of effortless attention to minute detail. His cuisine, original and astounding, is the expression of a philosophy based on natural farming and use of regional and seasonal ingredients. There is a transparency of flavor in his dishes which gives the sense that the the process of cooking continues within the elements of the food as it crosses the palate.

At table, Robert Rosellini is a samurai. Years of focussed attention to the elements of dining have left a pearl-like polish on every move and gesture. As his frequent dinner partner, I have felt strangely clumsy and uncertain as I noticed how perfectly the champagne and the appetizer seemed to finish precisely together just as the next dish was ready to be served. I had succumbed to the intoxication of the flavor and had destroyed my plate and emptied my glass much to quickly. In the presence of a master, one becomes more aware of one's unawareness.

I do not mean to give the impression that eating with Robert is a trial. On the contrary. It is exciting because there is so much to learn. He never demands anything of his guests, and the profundity of his own practice is invisible if you do not look for it. The highest power never needs to show itself.

In his presence, I have at times been able to borrow that awareness which allowed the Chinese cook to "not eat" his food. A clarity and vigor fills the mind, and course after course of fish, fowl, veal, venison, wild boar, punctuated by sorbets, salads concocted of wild greens and flowers, and a mesmerizing sequence of great, greater, greatest wines, followed by ports, brandies, and fine cigars is dematerialized without the anticipated impact on the body. It is mysterious and inexplicable; I only know that it has to do with a state of mind and not with digestion.

This introduction communicates only the tip of an iceberg. I invite you to enter Robert's world through his contribution to this book, and may the flavor of your life be forever enhanced.

Potage du Jour

Sable au Fenouil
(poached cape sable with fennel and cream)

ou Salade Tiede d'Agneau Sale
(warm salad of cured lamb and wild greens)

ou Pate d'Etes au Sauce de Groseilles
(summer pate of fresh herbs & cognac with gooseberry sauce)

Salade Impromptue
(Salad of local seasonal greens)

ou Granite de Peches et Hyssop
(Peach and anise hyssop ice)

Cabillaud aux Groseilles Sauvages (Braised rock cod with huckleberries)	19.00
Sole a la Creme d'Ecrivisses (poached fillet of sole with a rich crayfish sauce)	20.00
Papillote de Saumon au Vert d'Oseille (salmon fillet and fresh sorrel baked in a paper case)	20.00
Foie de Veau a la Moutarde (sauteed veal liver with mustard, demi glace and fresh bacon)	16.50
Cotes de Veau au Basilic (sauteed veal chop with fresh basil, veal stock and cream)	24.00
Demi Carre d'Agneau Roti aux Aromates (half a rack of lamb roasted with fresh aromatic herbs)	26.00
Boeuf a la Ficelle (fillet steak "on a string" with horseradish butter & marrow)	23.50
Pintadeau au Framboise (roast Guinea fowl with raspberries)	24.00

Les Fromages $4.50   Les Desserts from $2.00

The Last Word on Food and Dining

by Robert Rosellini

As a preliminary step toward clarity about diet as it related to food, you should master your body. I have no interest whatsoever in gaining or losing weight, however, or in wasting any time worrying about either one. Therefore, I leave the solution of how to achieve mastery of your body to each of you. I find dining to be too enjoyable for such an unproductive activity.

The only diet there is, is paying attention. Paying attention requires nothing. It requires only that you notice what food is there before you and enjoy it. The difficulty most diners have is that they do not pay attention. Their thoughts and ideas about food have already filled the space in which activity is taking place, and as a result, they have no opportunity to be there. Only their ideas are there. Because attempting to discover and clear the source of all these ideas about food could take a lifetime, you will find the quickest method is simply to focus your attention on what is actually on the plate. You will discover that you have nothing to fear from food and that you are the author of your body, not whatever you put into it. However, you will discover something that will initially present a problem—flavor.

The problem with flavor is that there is precious little of it to be found in what you eat. Flavor expressed through food can only be produced out of love. Flavor can not be produced out of trying to produce it or through any specific form of diet. The best method of securing flavor is to love your chef or whoever is preparing your meal.

Once you arrive at the level of paying attention and thus of noticing flavor, you will also discover that the nourishment you receive has little to do with the food you eat. Nourishment has more to do with your love of the chef and your ability to create a context in which to receive that love.

Perhaps some of what I am saying seems confusing. If so, then the next thought will not clear it up, but it will present an interesting opportunity to do so. If you pay too close attention to what you are eating, you will notice that it is not necessary to eat much at all. So why bother eating? Obviously, because dining itself is so much fun! The only diet there is, is love.

Final Thoughts

What I have learned, after years of research on myself, is that when I don't like part of my body and it is not the way I want it to be, that is where I am not letting God in. That is where I am resisting God. That is where I am stuck in my ego.

Think about it!

What if both underweight
AND overweight
were due to the same cause,
that of nourishing death
more than life?

*Nourish
your
life
urge!*

The Ultimate Nectar

The week before I finished this book I was standing in Jody's kitchen in Seattle describing to Robert the most divine taste in the world. I had had it once in Paris and I was wishing I could give it to him. At that very moment, my good friend Michele came over and heard this conversation. She said she had some and did we wish her to get it? I could not not believe my ears! It was a miracle.

There he was again. Saibaba. The Elixir of Immortality materialized right out of his body. Nothing sweeter on earth had I ever tasted! The Essence of the Divine, and I could have MORE? I had thought that the time in Paris was an experience to be had once in a lifetime. But who was I to put such a limiting thought around the Divine? Here it was coming to me again and immediately upon my asking! I was very humbled. Could it really be the same?

I decided on a ceremony. I woke up everyone in the house. Jack agreed to sing and play music. I got Jody out of bed. When Michele returned, she began to sing chants of Saibaba. We waited for the right moment. It was very holy, very holy indeed. She poured a drop into my hand. I said I hoped there was enough for everyone. How funny, now that I think of it, to say that of the Divine! My drop began to increase. It seemed alive. This Elixir of Immortality, Michele said, she had collected from a shrine in India where it dripped now and then out of his picture. I knew that what she said was true, even though I had never heard of the shrine before.

I licked the Elixir out of my palm. There could be no doubt. It was the same! One could never ever forget that taste, that moment. I licked it again. It increased until I had trouble believing what was happening. We were all speechless. We all melted into the floor. The others seemed to go into a deep stupor. Michele, who is my body therapist, began to massage my body. I could not feel a thing. I knew that my DNA was reorganizing. I knew my body was definitely going through a very big change. I knew that I had had total communion and I was forever blessed.

I can best describe that moment by sharing with you what I wrote to Saibaba after that experience.

O, Saibaba,
I ate everything
  But still hungered for God,
I drank everything
  But I still thirsted for God,
I touched everything
  But I still wanted to feel God,
I listened to everything
  But I still wanted to hear God.
  and then . . .
You came to me in Paris
  three years ago,
You came to me again
  in the volcano,
You came to me most recently in the kitchen
  and many other times I did not know.

I tasted your ash,
I drank your nectar,
  And I was finally nourished
  And I was finally satisfied.

Karen Kingston author of

Creating Sacred Space
with
Feng Shui

Clear Your Clutter with
Feng Shui

133.3
K

Free Yourself from
Physical Mental
Emotional and
and Spiritual Clutter

originally published in 1998 in
Great Britian by
Judy Piatkus (Publishers)
Limited.

Farewell

[handwritten notes:]

Feel the Fear and Do It Anyway
and
End the Struggle and
Dance with Life
Susan Jeffers' Books

Moving on from relationships
different paths divergent want

If you are really determined to solve your problem, I know you are willing to do anything to make that happen. You must be determined to see the truth about it. Seeing the truth about anything heals it. You must be willing to face the cause of your condition and the negative thoughts behind it. You have to be willing to give them up. It is like saying, "Get Thee behind me, Satan!" That is how Jesus took command. You, too, must take command of your mind.

Prayer is the most powerful way I have learned to do this. I gave up control and let God control my mind. I have found that this simple prayer ritual works for everything. If you want things to work for you, I suggest you try it. I have never found anything as powerful to bring *permanent and lasting results in healing* as the following ritual.

1. Change all your thoughts to the highest spiritual thoughts.
2. Use Rebirthing, giving up the birth trauma and other stuck negative mental mass through breathing.
3. Give up the death urge.
4. Pray and accept the atonement.

5. Love yourself.
6. Use the Ultimate Affirmation of Atonement.

I allow the Holy Spirit to undo all my wrong thinking that caused my problem and that keeps me stuck in this problem.

I surrender any problems I have about my body to the Holy Spirit.

I surrender the painful "payoff" I get from my problem to the Holy Spirit.

I surrender the attachment I have to my problem to the Holy Spirit.

I surrender the separation my problem gives me to the Holy Spirit.

I surrender the revenge I think I need that I get from my problem to the Holy Spirit.

I surrender my addiction to my problem to the Holy Spirit.

I surrender the way I use this problem to the Holy Spirit.

I surrender my need to use this problem as a weapon to the Holy Spirit.

I surrender to the Holy Spirit whatever it is that keeps me from letting it go completely.

I surrender my need to think and prove that God is an enemy.

I give up my fear of healing to the Holy Spirit.

OM NAMAHA SHIVA

(Lord Shiva, I bow before thee in Reverence. Please destroy my Ignorance.)

I cannot imagine any condition that could not be healed by this act. Please believe that I love you and I pray for your complete healing on this matter. In the name of Jesus, Babaji, Saibaba, Muktanana, and all the Avatars and Masters and my friends who have already mastered their lives. I ask that God release all of us from fear and the ego.

Love,

Sondra Ray!

DON'T Sweat the Small Stuff ... And It's all Small Stuff

became Rolfer deep massage technique emotional stuff comes out

Readers interested in obtaining additional information on Rebirthing or LRT should write the following addresses:

due art D.S.S. Stuff with your family
98

LRT
145 West 87th Street
New York, NY 10024
(212) 799-7323

To locate a rebirther in your area call:
(1-800) 641-4645
Leave your name, address and phone number.

ORDER NOW!

Sondra's tape
YOUR IDEAL RELATIONSHIP WITH YOUR BODY AND WEIGHT

Affirmations for losing weight with music in the background.

Send $12.50 (includes tax and postage) to:

Life Unlimited
8125 Sunset, 204-O
Fair Oaks, CA 95628
(916) 967-8442

Write for a free catalog of tapes, related books, and other products available.